T0293086

CONCISE GUIDE TO MEDICINAL APPLICATION IN PEDIATRICS

Translation of Xiao Er Yao Zheng Zhi Jue

Other Related Titles from World Scientific

The Yellow Emperor's Classic of Medicine — Essential Questions
Translation of Huangdi Neijing Suwen
edited by Jinghua Fu
translated by Mingshan Yang
ISBN: 978-981-3273-57-3

A History of Medicine in Chinese Culture
In 2 Volumes
by Boying Ma
ISBN: 978-981-3237-96-4 (set)
ISBN: 978-981-3237-97-1 (Vol. 1)
ISBN: 978-981-3237-98-8 (Vol. 2)

CONCISE GUIDE TO MEDICINAL APPLICATION IN PEDIATRICS

Translation of Xiao Er Yao Zheng Zhi Jue

Yi Qian

Translated by: Mingshan Yang

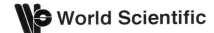

World Scientific

NEW JERSEY · LONDON · SINGAPORE · BEIJING · SHANGHAI · HONG KONG · TAIPEI · CHENNAI · TOKYO

Published by

World Scientific Publishing Co. Pte. Ltd.

5 Toh Tuck Link, Singapore 596224

USA office: 27 Warren Street, Suite 401-402, Hackensack, NJ 07601

UK office: 57 Shelton Street, Covent Garden, London WC2H 9HE

Library of Congress Cataloging-in-Publication Data
Names: Qian, Yi, author.
Title: Concise guide to medicinal application in pediatrics / Yi Qian,
    translated by Mingshan Yang.
Other titles: Xiao er yao zheng zhi jue. English
Description: New Jersey : World Scientific Publishing, [2020]
Identifiers: LCCN 2019034396 | ISBN 9789811207655 (hardcover)
Subjects: MESH: Pediatrics | Signs and Symptoms | Medicine, Chinese Traditional |
    Formularies as Topic | China
Classification: LCC RJ61 | NLM WZ 290 | DDC 618.92--dc23
LC record available at https://lccn.loc.gov/2019034396

British Library Cataloguing-in-Publication Data
A catalogue record for this book is available from the British Library.

B&R Book Program

《金匮要略方论译注·小儿药证直诀译注》
Originally published in Chinese by China Renmin University Press
Copyright © China Renmin University Press 2009
English translation rights arranged with China Renmin University Press

For any available supplementary material, please visit
https://www.worldscientific.com/worldscibooks/10.1142/11483#t=suppl

Desk Editor: Ling Xiao 萧玲

Typeset by Stallion Press
Email: enquiries@stallionpress.com

Printed in Singapore

Contents

About Qian Zhong Yang (Qian Yi)

by Liu Qi

Qian Yi, with styled name Zhongyang, was originally from Qiantang as ancestral home and was related to Wuyue King in ancient times. When Qian Chu (the King of Wuyue) dedicated his territories to the Song Dynasty, Qian Yi's grandfather Yun also followed him to go to the north and settled down in Yuncheng of Shandong. Qian Yi's father with his styled name Hao was good at acupuncture but addicted to alcohol and liked travelling. One day he concealed his identity and went to the east islands but since then he had not come back. Qian Yi's mother died when he was three years old; his aunt married a doctor surnamed Lv, and they adopted him as a son in sympathy. Qian Yi began to study and followed Mr. Lv to learn medicine after he grew up a little. When Mr. Lv was going to die, Mr. Lv told him about the details of his family; Qian Yi cried after listening and asked to look for his father's trace; through five or six journeys to and fro, he learned of his father's whereabouts at last. After a few more years, Qian Yi finally took his father back home when Qian Yi was more than 30 years old. The people in the village marveled at the matter and were moved to tears; many people wrote poems to praise it. Seven years later, his father died of old age, and Qian Yi held a funeral in accordance with local customs. Qian Yi served Mr. Lv as his own father; after Mr. Lv died, Qian Yi gave a burial and mourning to Mr. Lv because Mr. Lv had no sons; later Qian Yi helped to complete the marriage for Lv's daughter; moreover, Qian Yi held a ceremony to mourn Lv like his own father.

Initially Dr. Qian Yi was famous in Shangdong area for pediatric medicine. During Yuanfeng period, the daughter of the elder Princess (Emperor's sister) was ill and Dr. Qian was called in for treatment; he was offered the post of Hanlin Medical Officer and awarded crimson robes just because of the successful treatment of the daughter of the Princess. The next year, the master of Yiguo, the son of the Emperor, suffered from fright wind with convulsions, but the doctors in the palace failed to cure it. The elder Princess came to the palace, and talked about Dr. Qian Yi and said that he had a special ability although he was from a humble family. The Emperor called in Dr. Qian Yi immediately and Dr. Qian Yi cured the disease with *Huángtǔtāng* (黄土湯 *Terrae Flavae Decoction*). The Emperor summoned and praised him in public, and asked him why *Huángtǔtāng* (黄土湯 *Terrae Flavae Decoction*) could cure the disease. Dr. Qian Yi answered: "If earth dominates water, water will be calmed; liver wood can be balanced and symptoms of wind syndrome will be naturally stopped. Moreover, I just happened to treat the disease when it was almost going to heal because of the previous treatments by the other doctors." The Emperor was very happy to hear his answer and then promoted Dr. Qian as an Imperial Medical Officer and rewarded him with purple robes and goldfish bag as a token of imperial recognition. From then on, both the Royal courtiers and ordinary families were eager to seek medical help from him and Dr. Qian almost had no free days. When Dr. Qian lectured in medicine, few experienced doctors could beat him. Before long, Dr. Qian Yi quit the official position on the plea of illness. When the Zhezong Emperor ascended the throne, Dr. Qian was called again into the palace as an imperial doctor on duty. After a period of time, Dr. Qian asked for leave on the pretext that he was ill and Dr. Qian was no longer reinstated.

Dr. Qian Yi had a weak constitution by birth and forthright personality without paying attention to etiquette, and he was addicted to alcohol. He was affected by some diseases but he treated himself with his own understanding and resultantly his diseases were soon healed. When a serious disease attacked him late in the course, he was rather tired and then sighed: "This is the so-called general impediment syndrome. If general impediment involves the viscera, the patient would be dead; I am almost finished." After a while, he added: "I can move the evils away from my viscera to limbs." So he made the specific medicine by himself and drank it day and night, but nobody else had seen the formula. Before too long, he had contracture of his left hands and feet which made him disabled. Dr. Qian was happy to say: "That's OK." Then he sent his relatives to climb the Dong Mountain to inspect where *Túsī* (菟絲 *Chinese Dodder See*) grew; the relatives took lighted candles along and dug into the underground when the candle was blown out; they really obtained *Fúlíng* (茯苓 *Poria*) as big as a bucket. Then Dr. Qian Yi ate the *Fúlíng* according to a certain processing method and after a month the medicinal tuber was eaten up. From then on, although he was unable to move one half of his body, Dr. Qian's sinews and bones were as firm as a healthy person's. Later on, after he retreated and lived in seclusion, he didn't put on hat and shoes at home and sat or slept in bed; from time to time he read history books and any works available; when there were visitors, he had a free talk and drank with them. When he was in a good mood, he ordered two servants to carry him in a sedan chair up and down the streets. When people sometimes invited him to go out to visit, he refused it. Every day patients came for consultation, with some patients supported and some carrying a baby in the arms; his door was crowded with visitors seeking medical help. From the villages nearby to the places hundreds of miles away, usually there were people who came to see the doctor and they were all given medicine and left with grateful thanks.

One day, a princess royal (the daughter of the Emperor's sister) suffered from diarrhea and was going to die; Dr. Qian just got drunk when he was consulted and said: "She will certainly recover after eruption of rash." Douwei, the son-in-law of the princess didn't agree to it and angrily blamed him; Dr. Qian had no answer and went back. The next day, the princess developed a rash and was recovering; Douwei was very happy and wrote a poem to express his gratitude.

The son of the king living in royal Guangqin Palace was ill, and in consultation Dr. Qian said: "The disease can be cured without giving any medicine." Dr. Qian turned back to a younger child nearby and said: "The child will soon have a fulminant disease. After the noon on the third day, the child will be safe." The child's family angrily said: "What disease does the child have actually? The doctor scares us in order to covet interests." The next day the child developed epilepsy in urgent condition as expected and Dr. Qian was consulted again for treatment; after three days the child recovered. The family asked him: "Why could you predict the outcome before the child had illness?" Qian answered: "This child had surging fire and straightly staring eyes, indicating that his heart and liver were affected by evil. However, after noon the disease passed the due time when the heart and liver would develop illness."

There was a prince in the royal family, who suffered from diarrhea and vomiting; some doctors treated it with warm medicinals but the panting was getting worse. Dr. Qian Yi said: "The disease was affected by heat in origin and moreover spleen Qi was damaged; how can the drastic agent be used to dry it? Otherwise the patient will have no excretion. It is suitable to use *Shígāotāng* (石膏汤 *Gypsum Decoction*)." The king and other doctors didn't believe his words. After thanking, Dr. Qian retreated and said: "Please do not call me in again." After two days Dr. Qian was consulted again but Dr. Qian could not come in time because he just had something to do. The king was angry and suspected it as an excuse and then sent a dozen servants to urge. After arrival, Dr. Qian said: "It is indeed a syndrome of *Shígāotāng* (石膏湯 *Gypsum Decoction*)." Finally according to his order the treatment was really effective for the disease.

There was a scholar who suffered from cough, with pale and bluish complexion and difficult respiration. Dr. Qian Yi said: "This is due to liver wood retro-restraining lung, which is a reversal syndrome. If it occurs in the autumn, it is curable, but now it is in spring and the case is hopeless." The patient's family pleaded for medication and Dr. Qian reluctantly gave him some medicine. The next day, Dr. Qian said: "After taking two doses of medicine I gave you to purge liver fire, the disease hasn't subsided, and after invigorating lung but lung deficiency is getting worse; now the patient developed pale lips additionally and would die in three days. However if the patient can eat, he will survive the deadline but if he cannot eat, he will not survive the harsh time. Today the patient can still take some porridge, so he will live for more than three days." After five days, the patient died.

A pregnant woman was ill and some doctor claimed that her disease was rooted in the fetus which should be removed. Dr. Qian Yi said: "During pregnancy the fetus is maintained by providing nutrition through her five solid viscera and the cycle is completed for sixty days. If you can wait for the due month to nourish the corresponding viscera, why abort the fetus?" Later, both mother and child were saved.

There was a lactating woman who was ill because of great fear; she recovered but kept her eyes open and could not shut her eyes when sleeping. People didn't know the reason and went to consult Dr. Qian. Dr. Qian said: "*Yùlǐjiǔ* (鬱李酒 *Wine of Pruni Japonicae*) can be cooked for her to drink, and after drinking her disease will be cured. The reason for the therapy is that, the eyes are related with liver and gallbladder internally; if Qi is stagnated due to fright, gallbladder Qi is spreading transversely and doesn't go down smoothly. Only *Yùlǐ* (鬱李 *Pruni Japonicae*) can remove the stagnation which goes into gallbladder with wine; when the stagnation disappears, her eyes can open and close normally." According to the order of Dr. Qian, the disease was really cured.

One day, Dr. Qian visited Shanwen's house and was surprised by baby's crying; he asked: "Whose family had this baby's crying?" Shanweng answered: "This is the crying from my twin boys." Dr. Qian said: "Please take good care of your babies and in one hundred days their lives could be safe."

Shanwen was very unhappy at the time. After more than a month, the two boys died.

Dr. Qian Yi made prescriptions in medical practice with comprehensive consideration and did not stick to the theory of only one scholar; he could cure a variety of diseases and his skills were not only limited to pediatrics. He was well-versed in books available; when others adhered to the ancient books, Dr. Qianvyi could go beyond the previous fashion and his innovation could coincide with the ancient spirit wonderfully. He was well learned in material medica, for which he knew much about the innate laws of things and could differentiate the right from the wrong in the historical pharmaceutical works. If people sometimes took some rare medicinal herbs or had questions to ask for advice, Dr. Qian Yi could tell them the complete process of growth, where and when the herbs could be collected, and the quality and nomenclature; people found what he said was all correct according to the ancient works of pharmacy when they came back to have a check. With the impediment disease, Dr. Qian's symptoms of limbs spasm were getting worse in later years; unfortunately Dr. Qian did not give up his addiction to alcohol and cold food. He learned that his disease was incurable and he called in his family and relatives to bid farewell; Dr. Qian died at home at the age of eighty-two. Dr. Qian Yi wrote five volumes of *Careful Treatise of Cold-Damage* and 100 articles of *On Infant and Child*. A son of Qian Yi died early and his two grandsons are now working as doctors.

The author (Liu Qi) commented that Qianyi was famous for not only his medical skills but also other qualities, such as his sincere behavior like a Confucian scholar, his unusual integrity like a chivalrous person and his secluded life with high medical reputation like the moral person. He said to the author several times: "In the past, in order to study the theory of five phases and six seasonal Qi, I stayed at the top of Dongping King's mausoleum at night and observed the celestial phenomena for more than one month without sleeping. Now that I am getting old and going to die, I feel that there are many things not to be recorded in books indeed; can you follow me for thirty days and I will impart all my knowledge to you." I said with a smile: "Thank you for taking a fancy to me but I do not have enough time." After that, this matter had not been mentioned. Ah! It's too difficult to find a person like Qian Yi. After Qian Yi died, I heard that he had cured so many cases that his medical practice was eulogized by the people in Dongtai state. Now I select some outstanding medical records into this biography, which will serve as reference to historians to write biographies for the doctor.

List of Translators

Translator-in-Chief	Yang Mingshan	杨明山
Vice Translators-in-Chief	Liu Yuting	刘玉婷
	Jin Yong	晋 永
	Zhu Cui	朱 萃
Translators	Zhang Jun	张 俊
	Zhang Junlu	张君璐
	Kang Zhiran	康知然
	Yang Liang	杨 良
	Liu Shanshan	刘珊珊

Part I

1

The Method of Pulse-Taking for Young Children

小儿脉法

It is difficult to treat diseases with severely abnormal pulse; if Qi is not in harmony, the pulse will be stringy and swift; if the disease is caused by maldigestion, the pulse will be sunken and slow; if the disease belongs to deficient-fright, the pulse is irregular and swift; if the disease is due to wind, the pulse is floating and if the disease is due to cold, the pulse is sunken and thin.

2

Thriving Changes

变蒸

When a fetus is in the womb, it has grown in bone Qi, and five solid viscera and six hollow viscera have been formed but not developed fully. After birth, the baby grows in bone and vessels continually which are the soul of five solid viscera and six hollow viscera. So-called thriving changes are the positive development. The child in thriving changes develops from internal to external as well as from down to up, having much warm sense of the body; so at the 32nd day after birth, there is one thriving change. At the end of every thriving change, its mind and mood are different from before. What is it? In fact it grows and develops viscerally and intellectually. How about the growing bones and developing spirit? There are 365 bones; besides forty-five small bones, there are 320 bones. After birth, the bones grow ten sections upward within a day, that is, there are 100 sections within ten days and there are 320 sections within 32 days, which is termed one round and also termed a thriving change. The residual Qi of the bone divides from the brain into the gums and makes the 32 teeth. And there erupt teeth less than 32 because there are insufficient thriving changes compared with the norms. Or at the 28th day there erupt twenty-eight teeth, and the following shares the same rule but there will be no more than 32 in number. After one round, there will be deficient fever, which all infantile diseases tend to have. After ten rounds the small thriving change is finished. Within 320 days there grows bone Qi, which has the complete structure but not develops fully. So till 32nd day, there is the first thriving change, and kidney and mind develop. Till 64th day there is thriving change again and develops bladder with cold sense in ears and sacrococcyx. Both kidney and bladder govern water and water pertains to one in number, so they have thriving changes first. At 96th day after birth there is the third thriving change; at 128th day there develops small intestine, during which the infant has sweating and slight fright. Heart corresponds to fire and fire pertains two in number. Till 160th day there is the fifth thriving change, and liver is grown and the baby is capable of crying; at 192nd day there is the sixth thriving change and the bladder is grown, during which the eyes cannot open and appear reddish. Liver corresponds to wood and wood pertains to three in number. Till 224th day there is the seventh thriving change, and lung is grown and the baby is capable of making voice; at 256th day there is the eighth thriving change and the intestine is grown, during which the skin seems warm with or without sweating. The lung corresponds to metal and the metal pertains to four in number. Till 288th day there is the ninth thriving change and the spleen is grown with developing wisdom. Till 320th day there is the tenth thriving change and the stomach is grown, during which the baby tends to have anorexia, gut pain and milk reflux. Both spleen and stomach correspond to earth and earth pertains to five in number. Till then the thriving changes have completed. After then the teeth grow continually and the baby is capable of simple speech and knowing joy and anger, so it can be said that the thriving changes have been completed. Taicang stated that Qi will spread into four limbs and grows small bones within the ten thriving changes. After sixty-fourth day the meridians and vessels grow and hands and feet receive the blood, so the hand can hold things and the baby can walk. It is said in the classics that there are changes together with thriving, which can be regarded as thriving completeness and its timing is at one year old. The teacher said: For fever with no sweating, diaphoresis can be applied; for severe vomiting, the purgation can be slightly applied; any other therapies cannot be adopted in treatment. Therefore the baby should undergo the thriving changes. Loss of deciduous teeth is like moving sprout of the flower; so-called eruption with less than 32 teeth is caused by insufficiency thriving, because the tooth eruption should be in accord with the date of thriving change; after reaching adulthood, the number of teeth can be observed to reflect thriving changes clearly.

3

What the Five Viscera Govern

五脏所主

Heart governs fright. There are crying, fever and convulsions after drinking much water in its excessive syndrome; there are irritation and restlessness when sleeping in its deficient syndrome.

Liver governs wind. There are staring eyes, wailing, yawning, stiff nape and sudden stuffiness in its excessive syndrome; there are grinding teeth and frequent yawning in its deficient syndrome. With hot weather there happens external Qi, and with wet weather there happens internal Qi.

Spleen governs fatigue. There are drowsiness, body fever and drinking much water in its excessive syndrome; there are vomiting, diarrhea and limb convulsions in its deficient syndrome.

Lung governs panting. There are chest tightness and panting with or without drinking much water in its excessive syndrome; there are unsmooth breath and long inhalation in its deficient syndrome.

Kidney governs deficiency with no excessive syndrome. There are only sores and rashes; if kidney is excessive, the sores and rashes become black and depressed.

In particular the deficiency and excess of five viscera should be differentiated. If lung disease is complicated by the liver syndrome, there appear teeth grinding and frequent yawning, which are easy to be treated because deficient liver cannot dominate lung. If there are staring eyes, wailing, stiff nape and sudden stuffiness, the disease is difficult to treat. If lung disease lasts for a long term, there appears deficient cold and excessive liver retro-restrains lung. According to the conditions of the new or chronic as well as the deficient or excessive, the mother organ should be supplemented if it is deficient and the child-organ should be purged if it is excessive.

4

Diseases of Five Solid Viscera

五脏病

Liver disease: crying, stared eyes, yawning, sudden stuffiness and stiff nape.

Heart disease: frequent crying, fright, shaking of hands and feet, fever and polydipsia.

Spleen disease: drowsiness, diarrhea and no desire for food.

Lung disease: stuffiness, unsmooth breathing, long expiration, short of breath and panting.

Kidney disease: spiritless eyes, photophobia and heavy body bones.

5

Liver Affected by Exogenous Evil to Cause Wind

肝外感生风

If there are yawning, sudden stuffiness, hot breath from the mouth, it should be dispersed with *Dàqīnggāo* (大青膏 *Great Blue Paste*). If the child can have regular diet and drink water frequently, *Dàhuángwán* (大黄圆 *Rhubarb Pill*) should be given for mild purgation. For the other conditions, purgation is not allowed.

6

Liver Heat

肝热

If the child is seen to grope for the collar and grasp objects aimlessly, *Xièqīngyuán* (瀉青圓 *Purging Blue (Liver Fire) Pill*) is applied mainly. If the child has high fever, drinks much water, has panting and stuffiness, *Xièqīngyuán* (瀉青圓 *Purging Blue (Liver Fire) Pill*) is applied mainly.

7

Lung Heat

肺热

If the child is seen to rub the eyebrows, eyes, nose and face by hands, *Gānjútāng* (甘桔湯 *Decoction of Liquorice Root and Platycodon Root*) is applied mainly.

8

Lung Exuberance Complicated by Cold Wind

肺盛复有风冷

If there appear chest fullness, shortness of breath, dyspnea, panting and Qi surging, it should be first given dispersing lung Qi and then given dispelling cold evil of wind. To disperse lung Qi, *Xièbáisǎn* (瀉白散 *Purging White (lung heat) Powder*) and *Dàqīnggāo* (大青膏 *Great Green Paste*) are given mainly. If lung is only affected by cold evil, there appears no chest fullness.

9

Deficient Heat Due to Lung

肺虚热

If the child's lip color is dark red, it can be treated by dispersing deficient heat of lung and a small dosage of *Xièbáisǎn* (瀉白散 *Purging White (lung heat) Powder*) should be taken.

10

Deficient Damage of Lung

肺脏怯

If there appear pale lips, supplement lung Yin with *Ejiāosǎn* (阿膠散 *Donkey-Hide Gelatin Powder*). If there are chest fullness, rough breathing, panting and unsmooth breathing, it is difficult to treat because of damage of deficient lung.

Both spleen and lung diseases last for a long term and will cause deficiency and pale lips. Spleen is the mother-organ of lung; the mother-organ and child-organ cannot nourish mutually if both of them are deficient; the condition is termed "deficient damage of lung" which manifested in pale lips mainly; the lustrous pale lips suggest good prognosis and the pale lips like dead bone suggest death.

11

Heart Heat

心热

When sleeping, the child is found to have hot breath from the mouth or sleep in prone position as well as to have up-stretching and teeth grinding, all of which pertain to heart heat and *Dǎochìsǎn* (導赤散 *Redness (Heart Fire)-Purging Powder*) is applied mainly.

If there is hot heart-Qi, the child has hot feelings in heart and chest; because the child cannot express them verbally, he is prone to the cooling place so as to take the prone position when sleeping.

12

Heart Excess

心实

If there is excessive heart-Qi, the Qi will surge up but go down with difficulty; taking the prone position when sleeping, the child will have unsmooth breathing; thus the child prefers to take the prone position so that the Qi flow will be unobstructed up and down, for which *Xièxīntāng* (瀉心湯 *Decoction of Purging Heart Fire*) is applied mainly.

13

Kidney Deficiency

肾虚

Children have weak constitution innately, which is due to inadequate natural endowments, leading to deficiency of spiritual Qi. If there is much eye-white (sunset eyes), open fontanelle (no fontanelle closure) and pale compression, the child is difficult to be raised and he will live to no more than sixty-four years old. When the children grow up and are consumed by lust, most of them will live less than forty years old. Or the patient has kidney deficiency due to acquired diseases and has different mechanisms compared with the above. Moreover, the deficiency of kidney Qi leads to weakness of lower limbs, because the body bones are so heavy that the lower body cannot support. Kidney water is kidney essence and deficiency of kidney Yin leads to photophobia; it is better to adopt the method of supplementing kidney Yin mainly with *Dìhuángwán* (地黄圓 *Rehmaniae Pill*) in the treatment.

14

General Signs of Complexion

面上证

In complexion, the left cheek corresponds to liver, the right cheek corresponds to lung, the front head corresponds to heart, the nose corresponds to spleen and the chin corresponds to kidney. The child with red complexion indicates heat syndrome which can be treated according to the different correspondence.

15

Internal Signs of Eyes

目内证

If the eyes are reddish, it indicates hot syndrome of heart meridian, which is treated mainly with *Dǎochìsǎn* (導赤散 *Redness (Heart Fire)-Purging Powder*).

If the eyes are slightly reddish, it indicates deficient heat syndrome of heart meridian, which is treated mainly with *Shēngxīsǎn* (生犀散 *Powder of Raw Rhinoceros Horn*) .

If the eyes are greenish, it indicates heat syndrome of liver meridian, which is treated mainly with *Xièqīngyuán(Wán)* (瀉青圓 *Purging Blue (Liver Fire) Pill*). If the eyes are slightly greenish, it indicates liver deficiency, which is treated with supplementing therapy.

If the eyes are yellowish, it indicates hot syndrome of spleen and stomach meridian, which is treated mainly with *Xièhuángsǎn* (瀉黄散 *Powder of Purging (Yellow) Liver Fire*).

If there is no spirit in the eyes, it indicates deficiency of kidney essence, which is treated mainly with *Dìhuángwán* (地黄圓 *Rehmaniae Pill*).

16

Liver Disease
Retro-restraining Lung

肝病胜肺

Liver disease is often seen in autumn, because strong liver can retro-restrain lung while weak lung cannot dominate liver; it should be given to supplement both spleen and lung for treating liver. The mechanism of supplementing spleen is that strong mother-organ (spleen) can make child-organ excessive. To supplement spleen, *Yìhuángsǎn* (益黄散 *Benefiting Yellow* (*Spleen*) *Powder*) is applied; to treat liver disease, *Xièqīngyuán*(*Wán*) (瀉青圓 *Purging Blue* (*Liver Fire*) *Pill*) is applied mainly.

17

Diseased Lung Dominating Liver

肺病胜肝

Lung diseases are often seen in spring, because lung can dominate liver; it should be given to supplement kidney and liver for treating lung diseases. Feeble liver is very susceptible to diseases. To supplement liver and kidney, *Dìhuángwán* (地黄圓 *Rehmaniae Pill*) is applied; to treat lung diseases, *Xièbáisǎn* (瀉白散 *Purging White* (*lung heat*) *Powder*) is applied mainly.

18

Liver Generating Wind

肝有风

The child has frequent winking but no convulsions, and if being affected by heart heat additionally, the child will have convulsions. To treat liver (wind), *Xièqīngyuán(Wán)* (瀉青圓 *Purging Blue* (*Liver Fire*) *Pill*) is applied; to treat heart fire, *Dǎochìsǎn* (導赤散 *Redness* (*Heart Fire*)-*Purging Powder*) is applied mainly.

19

Liver Generating Heat

肝有热

The child has straight vision but no convulsions, and if being affected by heart heat additionally, the child will have convulsions. To treat liver (wind), *Xièqīngyuán(Wán)* (瀉青圓 *Purging Blue (Liver Fire) Pill*) is applied; to treat heart fire, *Dǎochìsǎn* (導赤散 *Redness (Heart Fire)-Purging Powder*) is applied mainly.

20

Liver Generating Wind Drastically

肝有风甚

The child has opisthotonos and limbs rigidity but no convulsions because heart is not affected by heat evil; it should be given to nourish kidney for treating liver disease. To nourish kidney, *Dìhuángwán* (地黄圆 *Rehmaniae Pill*) is given; to treat liver wind, *Xièqīngyuán* (瀉青圓 *Purging Blue (Liver Fire) Pill*) is applied mainly.

Whether it is a newly developed or chronic disease, they can all induce liver wind which stirs the head and eyes; eyes correspond to liver and when liver wind affects the eyes, it is as if wind is blowing up and down or right and left; though liver wind is moderate, the child cannot bear it, leading to frequent winking. If the heat invades the eyes and contacts the sinews and vessels, the two canthi will close tightly and the eyes cannot move flexibly, leading to staring eyes. If it is added with heart heat, there will develop convulsion, because both child- and mother-organ have excessive heat, in which wind and fire are struggling with each other. To treat liver (wind), *Xièqīngyuán* (瀉青圓 *Purging Blue (Liver Fire) Pill*) is applied; to treat heart fire, *Dǎochìsǎn* (導赤散 *Redness (Heart Fire)-Purging Powder*) is applied mainly.

25

21

Epilepsy with Convulsions

惊痫发搐

If the male child has convulsions, he will have left strabismus with no crying, and right strabismus with crying; If the female child has convulsions, she will have right strabismus with no crying, and left strabismus with crying. It is due to mutual domination (between lung and liver). Additionally the manifestations during attack should be considered.

22

Convulsions in the Morning

早晨发搐

Because of tidal fever, the child has high fever, upward strabismus, shaking of hands and feet, hot drooling from the mouth and stiff neck from three to nine in the morning. It is due to exuberant liver-fire and kidney should be nourished for treating liver diseases. To nourish kidney, *Dìhuángwán* (地黄圆 *Rehmaniae Pill*) is given; to treat liver diseases, *Xièqīngyuán(Wán)* (瀉青圓 *Purging Blue* (*Liver Fire*) *Pill*) is applied mainly.

23

Convulsions Around Noon

日午发搐

Because of tidal fever, the child has convulsions, fright, rest-lessness, upward strabismus, reddish sclera, lockjaw, drooling in the mouth and shaking of hands and feet from nine in the morning to three o'clock in the afternoon. It is due to exuber-ant heart-fire and should be treated by supplementing liver Yin and purging heart fire. To purge heart fire, *Dǎochìsǎn* (導赤散 *Redness* (*Heart Fire*)-*Purging Powder*) and *Liángjīngyuán* (涼驚圓 *Fright-Cooling Pill*) are applied mainly; to supplement liver, *Dìhuángwán* (地黄圓 *Rehmaniae Pill*) is given.

24

Convulsions Day and Night

日夜发搐

Because of tidal fever, the child has slight convulsions with panting, slight strabismus as well as ambiguous body fever, open eyes when sleeping, cold hands and feet with yellowish watery stool from three o'clock in the afternoon to nine o'clock at night. It is due to lung exuberance and should be treated by supplementing spleen and purging the fire of heart and liver. To supplement spleen, *Yìhuángsǎn* (益黄散 *Benefiting Yellow (Spleen) Powder*) is applied; to treat liver fire, *Xièqīngyuán(Wán)* (瀉青圓 *Purging Blue (Liver Fire) Pill*) is applied; to treat heart fire, *Dǎochìsǎn* (導赤散 *Redness (Heart Fire)-Purging Powder*) is applied.

25

Convulsions During the Night
夜间发搐

Because of tidal fiver, the child has mild slight convulsions accompanied by restless sleep, body fever, staring eyes, strabismus, phlegm in the throat, silvery or brownish stool, indigestion of milk and food, drowsiness and no desire for drinking water from nine o'clock at night, midnight untill one to three o'clock in the early morning. It should be treated by supplementing spleen and purging heart fire. To supplement spleen, *Xièhuángsǎn* (瀉黃散 *Powder of Purging Yellow (Liver Fire)*) is applied; to purge heart fire, *Dǎochìsǎn* (導赤散 *Redness (Heart Fire)-Purging Powder*) and *Liángjīngwán* (涼驚圓 *Fright-Cooling Pill*) are applied mainly.

26

Convulsions After Coryza

伤风后发搐

After coryza, the child has convulsions, hot breath from the mouth, yawning, sudden stuffiness and shaking of hands and feet. It should be dispersed with *Dàqīnggāo* (大青膏 *Great Green Paste*) mainly. Because the child has weak endowments and physique innately, he tends to have convulsions after the common cold.

27

Convulsions After Maldigestion

伤食后发搐

When the child has convulsions after maldigestion, he has body fever, excessive drooling, drowsiness or vomiting with anorexia and spasms. The treatment should be to arrest convulsions first, and after relief of convulsions, *Báibǐngzǐ* (白餅子 *Medicinal White Muffin*) is applied for purgation first and then *Ānshénwán* (安神圓 *Mind-tranquilizing Pill*) is applied.

28

Convulsions Within One Hundred Days After Birth

百日内发搐

With true (organic) convulsions, the child is doomed to death after no more than two or three paroxysms; with false convulsions, the conditions are not serious though occurring frequently. With true convulsions, there develops fright seizure internally; with false convulsions, the child is affected by exogenous cold wind. Because the blood and Qi are not full, the child cannot put up with the evil of cold wind, leading to convulsions. The evidence for recognizing the false convulsions is that there is hot breath from the mouth. It can be treated with dispersing method, mainly with *Dàqīnggāo* (大青膏 *Great Green Paste*) as well as *Túxìnfǎ* (塗囟法 *Therapy of Applying Paste over Fontane*) or *Yùtǐfǎ* (浴體法 *Medicinal Bath Therapy*).

29

Acute Seizure

急惊

The seizure will be triggered by loud noise or violent fright and the child will return to normal right after attack, because there is no damage of Yin essence in the body and it should be purged mainly with *Lìjīngyuán* (利驚圓 *Seizure-Relieving Pill*).

The child with acute seizure has original heat from hyperactive heart. There appear body fever, reddish complexion, thirst for water, hot breath from the mouth, yellow stool and brownish urine and even convulsions. As the exuberant heat will generate wind which corresponds to liver, the disease is associated with both exuberant Yang and deficient Yin, which is treated mainly with *Lìjīngyuán* (利驚圓 *Seizure-Relieving Pill*) to remove the phlegm-heat. The treatment cannot be combined with warm medicinals like *Bādòu* (巴豆 *Fructus Crotonis*), fearing for recurrent convulsions due to remaining deficient fever. The child is affected by phlegm-heat in heart and stomach and stirs to have convulsions when hearing the extraordinary noise. If there is extreme heat, the child will have spontaneous convulsions.

30

Chronic Seizure

慢惊

Due to vomiting and diarrhea or after illness, the child has deficient damage of spleen and stomach, and the manifestations include cold all over the body, also cold breath from mouth and nose, spasm of hands and feet sometimes, drowsiness and open eyes when sleeping; it is due to lack of spleen Yang, which is treated with *Guālóutāng* (栝蔞湯 *Trichosanthis Decoction*) mainly.

The difference of acute and chronic seizure is in the syndromes of Yin or Yang, which can be treated according to the differentiation. Acute seizure is suitably treated with cooling and purgation while chronic seizure is suitably treated with warm supplementation. In society many formulae have no such kind of differentiation and most of them delay the infantile disease. Moreover the child is affected by cold wind and has vomiting and diarrhea, which are considered spleen deficiency and treated with warm supplementation by many doctors; if not being cured, the doctors may treat it with cooling medicinals instead; if still not being cured, the doctors may consider it coryza in origin and then treat it with purgation casually; in fact when spleen Qi is deficient, it can be neither purged internally nor resolved externally; after more than ten days, the child develops drowsiness and open eyes when sleeping and body fever. Because there is wind evil in spleen and stomach, the stool cannot be shaped, leading to diarrhea; the wind evil in spleen should be removed and after wind evil regresses, the diarrhea will stop, which is treated with *Xuānfēngsǎn* (宣風散 *Wind-Dispersing Powder*). Later *Shǐjūnzǐyuán* (使君子圓 *Fructus Quisqualis Pill*) is applied to supplement stomach. Nevertheless the long-term vomiting and diarrhea are not cured and deficient spleen will generate wind and progress to chronic seizure.

31

Five Kinds of Epilepsy

五痫

The treatment for five kinds of epilepsy varies with the solid viscera concerned. Each solid viscus corresponds to an animal, which is treated with *Wǔsèwán* (五色圓 *Five Colors Pill*).

Canine-like epilepsy: there are opisthotonos, upward stretching and crying like dog; these manifestations are associated with liver.

Sheep-like epilepsy: there are staring eyes, wagging tongue and crying like sheep; these manifestations are associated with heart.

Ox-like epilepsy: there are straight vision, abdominal distention and crying like ox; these manifestations are associated with spleen.

Rooster-like epilepsy: there are jerking due to fright, opisthotonos, spasm of hands and crying like rooster; these manifestations are associated with lung.

Pig-like epilepsy: the body is like a corpse and the child has white foamy saliva and cries like a pig; these manifestations are associated with pig.

For any type of epilepsies, the child with severe case will die and will also die if the epilepsy is getting more and more severe.

32

The Manifestations of Pox and Rash

疮疹候

The manifestations of dry face, reddish cheeks, also red eye-lids, yawning, sudden stuffiness, alternate cold and fever, cough, sneeze, cold tips of fingers and toes, restlessness and drowsiness when sleeping at night complicate the syndrome of pox and rash, which is termed epidemic disease. Only warm and cool medicinals can be used for the treatment; frenetic purgation and dispersion are not allowed and the cold wind should be avoided.

For this epidemic disease, there is a special sign attributed to five solid viscera respectively: blister attributed to liver, pustule attributed to lung, macules attributed to heart, rash attributed to spleen and black-turning spot attributed to kidney. Only after macular rash develops, it is possible to progress to epilepsy while the other types of pox are not prone to epilepsy. Wood (liver) restrains (earth) spleen just because wood (liver) contributes to (fire) heart. If it is the cold convulsions, *Liángjīngyuán(wán)* (凉驚圆 *Fright-Cooling Pill*) can be applied; if it is warm convulsions, *Fěnhóngyuán(wán)* (粉紅圓 *Warmly-Relieving-Seizure Pill*) can be applied.

When the fetus grows in the womb for ten months, it will take in the turbid blood from maternal five solid viscera and the maternal toxin will emerge after birth; so the manifestations of pox and rash all contribute to the fluids of five solid viscera. Liver governs tears, lung governs snivels, heart governs blood and spleen governs the control of blood circulation. Therefore there are five types of pox: the blister attributed to liver has watery issue like tears with bluish and small spot; the pustule attributed to the lung has issue like thick and turbid snivels with whitish and large spot; because the heart governs blood, the macule attributed to the heart has issue with reddish and small spot smaller than blisters; the rash attributed to the spleen has smaller spot than macule, and spleen governs blood circulation, so the rash has light reddish and yellowish color. Because the snivels and tears tend to have large amount, the pustules and blisters are relatively large. Since the blood nourishes the internal and flows out slightly, the macular rashes are relatively small. A child with blisters and pustules has fewer snivels and tears, as if the bladder filled with water would become shriveled after water flows out.

In over three days after the onset of tidal fever, the heat evil spreads into the skin and immediately the pox and rashes erupt; if there is not much eruption, it is because the heat evil lingers between the skin and interstitial striae. Tidal fever varies with the condition of solid viscera, e.g. lasting fever during the breakfast is regarded as blisters attributed to liver.

When the pox and rash develop, there appear the signs attributed to solid viscera except kidney, and only the general manifestations can be seen, including cold feeling of sacrococcyx and ears. Both sacrococcyx and ears correspond to kidney and to the north in direction, which governs the cold. If the pox appears black and sunken and the ears and sacrococcyx feel hot instead, it is a reversal syndrome. If *Bǎixiángyuán* (百祥圓 *Hundred-Luck Pill*) or *Niúlǐgāo* (牛李膏 *Paste of Radix Seu Cortex Rhamnus utilis*) is taken but there is no cure after taking three doses of each, it indicates the fatal disease.

When pox and rash develop, the severity can be judged according to the eruptive condition. When the pox and rash spread over the body immediately after eruption, it must be the severe condition; the eruption of pox accompanied by rash indicates the half serious and half light condition; sparse eruption indicates the mild condition. If the outer and inner parts are reddish and swollen, it indicates the mild condition; the black outer and red inner parts indicate slightly severe, and the white outer and black inner parts indicate the rather severe condition. If there is a black spot on the pox top like a pinhole, it indicates the drastically severe condition. If there appears purple, dry and sunken pox, with lethargy, profuse sweating, irritability, fever, thirst, abdominal distention, crying, panting and retained excretion, it indicates the extremely severe condition. When the child suffers from pox and rash, the lactating woman should pay more attention to diet and the child should avoid hunger and cold wind. Otherwise the evil will regress to kidney to make pox and rash turn black, which is difficult to treat.

The child with high fever should be treated by promoting urination; with low fever, the child should be given detoxification. The child having black, purple, dry and sunken pox and rash should be given *Bǎixiángyuán* (百祥圓 *Hundred-Luck*

Pill) for purgation; with non-black pox and rash, purgation is cautiously not allowed. Moreover, the severity should be judged according to the season and month concerned: generally pox and rash correspond to Yang, and the eruptive condition indicates compliance; so the disease occurring in spring and summer indicates compliance, and in autumn and winter, indicates reversal. Because in the winter months the kidney Qi is accordingly exuberant and the weather is extremely cold, the evil of the disease will regress to kidney and the pox and rash turn black. Additionally exanthem should be differentiated: pustule in spring, black sunken spot in summer, macule in autumn and rash in winter, all of which are also reversal but four or five in ten severe cases can survive. For the case with black spot, whenever it occurs, it is difficult for one in ten to survive. The manifestations include rigor and teeth chattering, or yellowish body and swollen and pink skin, which is better to be given *Băixiángyuán*(*wán*) (百祥圓 *Hundred-Luck Pill*). If the child fears cold continuously and feels body cold with profuse sweating but hot feeling of ears and sacrococcyx, it indicates the fatal disease. Why? Because the kidney Qi is so exuberant that the deficient spleen cannot restrain it. After purgation, the child has warm body and warm breath from the mouth with desire for drinking water, which can be treated; because spleen (earth) restrains kidney (water), the cold has been dispelled and the child feels warm. It is better to detoxicate the toxin in the treatment but frenetic purgation is not allowed, and otherwise the internal deficiency will drive the evil into kidney. If the child can have regular diet with charred scab on the top of pox and rash or has panting and constipation with non-black pox and rash, the purgation can be adopted. If there is body fever, vexing thirst, abdominal distention with panting, difficult excretion, reddish face, restlessness and heavy vomiting, urination should be promoted; if not being cured, it is better to apply *Xuānfēngsǎn* (宣風散 *Wind-Dispersing Powder*) for purgation. If the pox and rash do not form charred scab, it is caused by internal heat which is steaming in the skin so that the pox cannot form charred scab in 5–7 days after onset. It is better to apply *Xuānfēngsǎn* (宣風散 *Wind-Dispersing Powder*) together with *Shēngxī Mózhī* (生犀磨汁 *Wet-Grinding of Raw Rhinoceros Horn*) for detoxification and preventing heat, so that the pox and rash must form scab.

The mechanism of pox and rash is due to the successive domination of five solid viscera internally and only macule can cause convulsions. The rash is associated with the spleen, and if spleen is deficient, the liver will over-restrain it. Wood is going to dominate earth, and heat Qi will attack heart and mind that stir the spirit restlessly, so that the convulsions can progress to epilepsy. The macule is associated with heart that generates heat that generates wind that pertains to liver, and then the two viscera struggle and accordingly wind and fire conflict with each other, so that the convulsions will develop. In the treatment it should be prescribed to purge heart and liver and supplement the mother organ, including *Guālóutāng* (栝蔞湯 *Decoction of Fructus et Semen Trichosanthis*) as the main therapy.

The black pox and rash accompanied by acute diarrhea and bloody purulent stool with pox scab indicates compliance while indigestion of water and grain indicates reversal. Why? The black pox and rash are associated with the kidney because of innately strong spleen or previously supplemented spleen, so spleen Qi becomes exuberant and spleen can restrain kidney when kidney acts. Now the evil of pox and rash spreads into the abdomen and the scab forms, which shows that spleen is strong and kidney is regressing, that is, the evil of the disease is dispelled and then the life is safe. The etiology of indigestion of grain as well as milky diarrhea is that deficient spleen cannot restrain kidney, so that spontaneous diarrhea will happen, which must be difficult to treat.

33

Coryza

伤风

There are drowsiness, hot breath from the mouth, yawning and sudden stuffiness, which should be treated by dispersing heat evil with *Dàqīnggāo* (大青膏 *Great Green Paste*). If not being dispersed and there is indication for purgation, it should be purged with *Dàhuángwán* (大黄圆 *rhubarb Pill*). If the child drinks plenty of fluid and has a good appetite, it can be treated with slight purgation but it is not allowed for other types.

34

Cold Hands and Feet Due to Coryza

伤风手足冷

If spleen is feeble, harmonize spleen and later use disperse therapy. To harmonize spleen, *Yìhuángsǎn* (益黄散 *Benefiting Yellow (Spleen) Powder*) is applied; to disperse, *Dàqīnggāo* (大青膏 *Great Green Paste*) is applied.

35

Coryza Accompanied by Diarrhea

伤风自利

If spleen is deficient and feeble, supplement spleen with *Yìhuángsǎn* (益黄散 *Benefiting Yellow Powder*) and later disperse wind evil with *Dàqīnggāo* (大青膏 *Great Green Paste*). If not cured, *Tiáozhōngyuán* (調中圓 *Middle-Regulating Pill*) is applied mainly. If there is indication of purgation, *Dàhuángyuán(wán)* (大黃圓 *Rhubarb Pill*) followed by *Wēnjīngyuán* (溫驚圓 *Warmly-Relieving-Seizure Pill*) can be prescribed.

36

Abdominal Distention Due to Coryza

伤风腹胀

If spleen is deficient, spleen should be supplemented first; when panting completely disappears, disperse wind evil and then supplementation of spleen is still needed. To remove abdominal distentation, *Tāqìyuán* (塌氣圓 *Distention-Bleeded Pill*) is applied; to disperse wind evil, *Dàqīnggāo* (大青膏 *Great Green Paste*) is applied.

37

Coryza Involving Solid Viscera

伤风兼脏

If coryza involves heart, there appears palpitation due to fright; if lung is involved, there appear restlessness, panting, stuffiness with long exhalation and cough; if kidney is involved, there appears photophobia. Each syndrome mentioned above can be treated with the therapy of supplementing mother-organ because all these syndromes result from the deficiency of the solid viscera involved.

38

Residual Fever After Purgation for Coryza

伤风下后余热

If the child has overdose of purgative medicinals, there is deficient heat in the stomach and thirst but with less desire for water. It should be treated by enriching fluid in the stomach with more *Báizhúsǎn* (白术散 *Powder of Rhizoma Atractylodis Macrocephalae*).

39

The Same and Different Manifestations Between Cold-Damage and Pox-Rash

伤寒疮疹同异

With cold-damage, the male child has heavy body and sallow complexion; the female child has reddish complexion and panting and fears cold. There are hot breath from the mouth, yawning, sudden stuffiness and stiff nape in both male and female patients. If the child has pox and rash, there appear reddish cheek, vexation, profuse sneezing, palpitation, lethargy and cold limbs. For cold-damage, the dispersing therapy should be given, and for pox, the warm and moderate medicinals are used. For high fever, the therapy of detoxification is given. Other conditions can be treated referring to the previous descriptions.

40

Vomiting and Diarrhea with High Fever in the First Three Days After Birth

初生三日内吐泻壮热

The newborn with no desire for milk has indigested milk in stool or whitish stool, which indicates maldigestion; it should be treated by purging the food retention and later harmonizing stomach. For purgation, *Báibǐngzǐ* (白餅子 *Medicinal White Muffin*) is applied and for harmonizing stomach, *Yìhuángsǎn* (益黄散 *Benefiting Yellow (Spleen) Powder*) is applied.

41

The Newborn at the Age of Three to Ten Days After Birth Has Vomiting and Cool Body

初生三日以上至十日吐泻身温凉

If the newborn has no desire for milk and has bluish and whitish stool and indigestion of milk, it is the syndrome of upper-excess and lower-deficiency. Also there are complicated syndromes: Involving lung — open eyes when sleeping and panting; involving heart — palpitation due to fright and thirst for drinking water; involving spleen — lethargy and sleepiness; involving liver — yawning and sudden stuffiness; involving kidney — the child has no strength to speak and has photophobia. Purgation should be given and for complicated conditions involving solid viscera, supplement spleen with *Yìhuángsǎn* (益黄散 *Benefiting Yellow (Spleen) Powder*). The two syndromes often occur in autumn and summer.

42

The Newborn Has Vomiting

初生下吐

After the newborn is delivered, the dirt in the mouth should be wiped away; if the dirt is not wiped away, it will be swallowed in the throat to cause vomiting, which is treated mainly with *Mùguāyuán* (木瓜圓 *Pill of Common Floweringqince Fruit*). When the newborn is delivered, the mouth must be wiped clean. Otherwise the dirt will be swallowed down as soon as the newborn cries out and it will cause many kinds of diseases.

43

Vomiting and Diarrhea with Body Heat After Coryza

伤风吐泻身温

The child has alternative feelings of cold and fever, drowsiness, rough breath, yellowish and whitish stool, vomiting, indigestion of milk and cough sometimes. Also there is the complication involving five solid viscera. It should be given decoction of the monarch-like and minister-like medicinals with dissolved *Dàqīnggāo* (大青膏 *Great Green Paste*) and later given *Yìhuángsǎn* (益黄散 *Benefiting Yellow (Spleen) Powder*). If previously having medication of purgation or no indication of purgation, the therapy mentioned above is not allowed as caution. It is due to spleen and lung affected by cold to cause poor eating.

44

Vomiting and Diarrhea with Feverish Body After Coryza

伤风吐泻身热

The child sleeps a lot, has appetite for milk, drinks water constantly, spits sputum, and has yellowish watery stool, all of which are due to deficient heat of stomach leading to vomiting and diarrhea. The treatment should be to enrich fluid of stomach to prevent thirst and later dispersing medicinals should be given. To prevent thirst, *Báizhúsǎn* (白术散 *Powder of Rhizoma Atractylodis Macrocephalae*) is applied mostly; to disperse heat and relieve exterior, *Dàqīnggāo* (大青膏 *Great Green Paste*) is applied.

45

Vomiting and Diarrhea with Cool Body After Coryza

伤风吐泻身凉

The child has white foaming saliva, diarrhea with bluish and whitish stool, stuffiness, no thirst, long exhalation after unsmooth exhalation and open eyes when sleeping; because the coryza subsides very slowly and the child has feeble constitution, it results in vomiting and diarrhea. The treatment should be to supplement spleen and later to disperse heat evil. To supplement spleen, *Yìhuángsǎn* (益黄散 *Benefiting Yellow (Spleen) Powder*) is applied; to disperse heat and relieve exterior, *Dàqīnggāo* (大青膏 *Great Green Paste*) is applied. The two syndromes often occur in spring and winter.

46

Similarity of Tidal Fever and Exuberant Fever Due to Wind-Heat

风温潮热壮热相似

The tidal fever begins at a certain time and subsides after the due time; the next day the tidal fever recurs in the same manner, which indicates the approaching seizure. The high fever has a high plateau and even progresses to epilepsy. The child with wind-heat syndrome has body fever and hot breath from the mouth as well as manifestations due to wind syndrome. The child with moderate heat syndrome feels warm but has no fever.

47

Similarity Between Aphonia and Dysphonia Due to Feeble Kidney

肾怯失音相似

After vomiting and diarrhea or a serious illness, the child cannot speak out though is able to produce vocal sounds and also swallow. It is not aphonia but because kidney Yin is too deficient to connect (heart) Yang. The treatement should be to supplement kidney with *Dìhuángyuán(wán)* (地黃圓 *Rehmaniae Pill*). Aphonia is just an acute disease.

48

Similarity for Yellowish Pigmentations

黄相似

If there is yellowish color over the body, skin and eyes, this is termed yellow disease. If there are body pain, stiff shoulder and neck, unsmooth excretion, yellowish body, yellowish face, eyes and nails, dark urine with color like house dust, predominance of yellow color in vision and thirst, this is difficult to treat and called jaundice. The two syndromes occur mostly after a serious illness. There is another syndrome with slight yellowing over the body which does not occur after illness but in fact is associated with stomach heat. The same is true of adults. Also, there is yellowish face, bulging abdomen, involuntary ingestion of soil and thirst, which is the chronic malnutrition of spleen. Moreover, there is yellowish pigmentation of the body after birth, which is termed neonatal jaundice. It is said in ancient medical books that all kinds of jaundice belong to heat syndrome with dark yellow color over the body. If there is sallow body with whitish color, it is due to feeble stomach and disharmony of stomach.

49

Vomiting and Diarrhea in Summer and Autumn

夏秋吐泻

After the 15th day of the fifth lunar month, the child may have vomiting, diarrhea and hot feeling of body and abdomen, which is due to excessive heat. Among the viscera involved, nine in ten are in hot condition. Or the child affected by hot milk has vomiting, indigestion of milk and diarrhea with dark yellow stool, which is treated mainly with *Yùlùsǎn* (玉露散 *Jade-Dew Powder*).

After the 15th day of the sixth lunar month, the child may have vomiting, diarrhea and a little hot feeling of body; among the viscera involved six in ten are in hot condition and four in ten in cold condition. The child has vomiting, indigestion of milk, diarrhea with yellow and whitish stool, a little thirst with or without appetite for milk. Before feeding, slight dosage of *Yìhuángsǎn* (益黄散 *Benefiting Yellow Powder*) is given and after feeding more dosage of *Yùlùsǎn* (玉露散 *Jade-Dew Powder*) is given.

After the seventh day of the seventh lunar month, the child may have vomiting, diarrhea and cool feeling of body; among the viscera involved three in ten are in hot condition while seven in ten are in cold condition. The child cannot take milk and has lethargy, restlessness, sudden stuffiness with long exhalation, open eyes when sleeping, pale lips, frequent retching and more sense to retch but no thirst. Before feeding, slight dosage of *Yìhuángsǎn* (益黄散 *Benefiting Yellow Powder*) is given and after feeding more dosage of *Yùlùsǎn* (玉露散 *Jade-Dew Powder*) is given.

After the 15th day of the eighth lunar month, the child may have vomiting, diarrhea and cold body, indicating Yang deficiency. The child has no appetite for milk, retching and diarrhea with bluish and brownish watery stool. Spleen should be supplemented mainly with *Yìhuángsǎn* (益黄散 *Benefiting Yellow Powder*) and purgation is not allowed.

50

Vomiting Milk

吐乳

There is vomiting milk and diarrhea with yellowish stool, which is due to feeding of hot milk; there is vomiting milk and diarrhea with bluish stool, which is due to feeding of cold milk. Both of them are treated with purgative therapy.

51

Deficiency and Emaciation

虛羸

Disharmony of spleen and stomach leads to no appetite for milk which results in emaciation. Also after severe illness or vomiting and diarrhea, spleen and stomach are weak and not capable of transporting and digesting grain Qi. The child with cold type of deficiency and emaciation has diarrhea often with bluish and whitish lips and mouth; the child with hot type of deficiency and emaciation has moderate body fever and yellowish skin and muscles. These are cold and hot types of deficiency and emaciation. For the cold type, *Mùxiāngyuán* (木香圓 *Costusroot Pill*) is mainly applied but not allowed in summer months; however, if there is indication concerned, slight dosage of *Mùxiāngyuán* (木香圓 *Costusroot Pill*) can be applied. For the hot type, *Húhuángliányuán* (胡黃連圓 *Pill of Rhizoma Picrorhizae*) is mainly applied but not allowed in winter months; however, if there is indication concerned, slight dosage of *Húhuángliányuán* (胡黃連圓 *Pill of Rhizoma Picrorhizae*) can be applied.

52

Coughing

咳嗽

Cough is often caused by slight cold evil affecting lung. In the eighth and ninth lunar months, lung Qi is exuberant, so coughing then must be excessive but is not a chronic disease. The manifestations include reddish face, profuse sputum and body fever and it should be treated with *Tínglìyuán* (葶藶圓 *Papergrass Seed Pill*). If lasting for a long time, it is not allowed to apply purgative therapy. Cough occurring in the 11th and 12th lunar months is often due to coryza. The wind evil invades Feishu acupoint (BL13) on the third thoracic vertebra and it should be given *Máhuángtāng* (麻黃湯 *Decoction of Chinese Ephedra Herb*) mainly for diaphoresis. The manifestations of heat syndrome include reddish face, thirst for water, hot spittle and sore throat and it is better to apply *Gānjútāng* (甘桔湯 *Decoction of Liquorice Root and Platycodon Root*) in the treatment. Till the fifth or seventh day, the cough syndrome has manifestations in body fever and spitting viscous saliva, which are treated with *Biǎnyínyuán* (褊銀圓 *Flat Mercury Pill*). If there exist exuberant lung Qi, cough followed by panting, body fever, and puffy face with thirst for water or without thirst, *Xièbáisăn* (瀉白散 *Purging White Powder*) is used for purgation. If the cough due to coryza lasts from five to seven days, and there is no hot syndrome but only cough, it is treated with *Tínglìyuán* (葶藶圓 *Papergrass Seed Pill*) for purgation and later with medicinals for resolving phlegm. If there is lung deficiency, and the child has cough, sudden stuffiness and then long exhalation frequently and noise in the throat, this is a chronic disease and should be treated with *Ejiāosăn* (阿膠散 *Donkey-Hide Gelatin Powder*) for supplementation. For profuse sputum, the treatement is first to supplement spleen and later *Biănyínyuán* (褊銀圓 *Flat Mercury Pill*) is given for slight purgation; lung is supplemented as soon as the drooling subsides and the therapy for supplementing lung is the same as in the previous description. For cough with vomiting clear water or greenish water, *Băixiángyuán* (百祥圓 *Hundred-Luck Pill*) is applied mainly. For cough with spitting spittle and milk, *Báibĭngzĭ* (白餅子 *Medicinal White Muffin*) is applied for purgation. If there is cough with expectoration of pus and blood, it is due to lung heat syndrome and the child can take *Gānjútāng* (甘桔湯 *Decoction of Liquorice Root and Platycodon Root*) after feeding. For chronic cough due to loss of lung liquid, *Ejiāosăn* (阿膠散 *Donkey-Hide Gelatin Powder*) is applied for supplementation. For cough with slight excessive phlegm, panting, red face with thirst for water sometimes, the child is treated with *Biănyínyuán* (褊銀圓 *Flat Mercury Pill*) for purgation. The main principle for treating cough is as follows: purgation for exuberant evil, supplementation for chronic course, and differentiation of deficiency and excess in order to add or reduce ingredients.

53

Various Infantile Malnutrition

诸疳

Infantile malnutrition in the internal manifests in swollen eyes, abdominal distention, diarrhea with changable colors of stool or with bluish and whitish forming stool and gradual emaciation; this is cold infantile malnutrition.

Infantile malnutrition in the external manifests in red ulcer below the nose and involuntary scratching; at the apex of the nose there is sore without encrustation usually, which infiltrates around ears. In the treatment of nasal sore and ulcer, *Lánxiāngsǎn* (蘭香散 *Herbaseu Radix CaryopteridisIncanae Powder*) is applied. For other sores, *Báifěnsǎn* (白粉散 The Whites Powder) is applied.

Infantile malnutrition associated with liver manifests in white nebula covering eyeballs and the treatement should be to nourish liver Yin mainly with *Dìhuángyuán(wán)* (地黄圓 *Rehmaniae Pill*).

Infantile malnutrition associated with heart manifests in sallow complexion, red cheek and high body fever, and the treatment should be to supplement heart mainly with *Ānshényuán(wán)* (安神圓 *Mind-Tranquilizing Pill*).

Infantile malnutrition associated with spleen manifests in sallow body, bulging abdomen and involuntary ingestion of soil; the treatment should be to supplement spleen mainly with *Yìhuángsăn* (益黄散 *Benefiting Yellow (Spleen) Powder*).

Infantile malnutrition associated with kidney manifests in emaciation as well as sores and scabies in the body, and the treatment should be to nourish kidney mainly with *Dìhuángyuán(wán)* (地黄圓 *Rehmaniae Pill*).

Infantile malnutrition associated with sinew manifests in diarrhea with bloody stool and emaciation, and the treatment should be to supplement liver mainly with *Dìhuángyuán(wán)* (地黄圓 *Rehmaniae Pill*).

Infantile malnutrition associated with lung manifests in panting and sores on the mouth and nose, and the treatment should be to supplement spleen and lung mainly with *Yìhuángsăn* (益黄散 *Benefiting Yellow (Spleen) Powder*).

Infantile malnutrition associated with bone manifests in preference to sleep on the cold ground and the treatment should be to nourish kidney with *Dìhuángyuán(wán)* (地黄圓 *Rehmaniae Pill*).

For any types of infantile malnutrition, the treatment should be based on the proper viscus involved and the principle that the mother-organ should be supplemented if it is deficient, as well as the selection of medicinals for treating infantile malnutrition; the cold type should be treated with *Mùxiāngwán* (*Costusroot Pill*) mainly while the hot type should be treated with *Húhuángliányuán(wán)* (胡黄連圓 *Pill of Rhizoma Picrorhizae*) mainly.

All the infantile malnutritions belong to the diseases of spleen and stomach and are caused by loss of liquid and fluid. After a serious disease or vomiting and diarrhea, the patient is treated with emetic for purgation, which will make spleen and stomach weak and cause loss of liquid and fluid. So the infantile malnutritions among young children are mainly iatrogenic diseases by foolish doctors. For example, tidal fever is associated with deficiency of one organ and excess of another organ, and deficient fever originates from the internal. Through supplementing mother-organ while purging the organ involved, the disease can be cured. If there is tidal fever at noon, it is deficient fever of heart; because liver is the mother-organ of heart, it is better to supplement liver first; when liver Qi is substantial, deficient fever of heart can be purged; after heart receives Qi from the mother-organ, deficient fever can be calmed down and tidal fever can be cured. Some doctors, meeting the case with tidal fever, wrongly consider it as excess syndrome and purge it with cold medicinals like *Dàhuáng* (大黃 *Radix Et Rhizoma Rhei*) and *Mǎyáxiāo* (馬牙硝 *Natrii Sulfas*). However, if giving too much purgation, the spleen and stomach will lose their controlling ability and the liquid and fluid will be exhausted, leading to infantile malnutrition. Taking aggregation as another example, it tends to cause attack with alternative chill and fever, thirst for water, and shaped hard lump below hypochondrium. It is treated with dispersing method gradually but some doctors reversely purge it with *Bādòu* (巴豆 *Fructus Crotonis*) and *Náoshā* (硇砂 *Sal Ammoniac*). Young children are susceptible to deficient or excessive syndrome, and if undue purgation is given, liquid and fluid in the stomach will be exhausted to cause infantile malnutrition leading to emaciation.

As to the disease of cold-damage, there is indication of purgation on the fifth or sixth day of the course; however, if too much cold medicinals are used, the liquid and fluid of spleen and stomach are getting scarce; even though the patient drinks water continuously, the deficient fever emerges internally. The hot Qi consumes liquid and fluid internally and the muscle is emaciated externally; if affected by other evils, the manifestations are complicated, leading to infantile malnutrition.

As to long-term vomiting and diarrhea or purgation wrongly given by some doctors, the deficient Qi will become worse and the liquid and fluid will be dried and damaged, which can also cause infantile malnutrition.

As to infantile malnutrition due to fatty food, it is also termed infantile malnutrition of spleen and its clinical pictures include thin and sallow body, dry skin as well as sores and scabies; its various manifestations include different symptoms and signs and here are a few typical ones: dry and unsmooth eyes, white nebula on the eyeballs, reddish lips, dry and sallow or blackish body, preference to sleep on the cold ground, involuntary ingestion of soil, scabies on the body, diarrhea with various colored feces like bluish, whitish and yellowish forming ones, proneness to bulging abdomen, sores over body, ears and nose, thin hair like tassel, big head with thin neck and body and thirst for water, etc, all of which are the manifestations concerned.

Generally, infantile malnutritions should be differentiated in terms of cold and hot as well as fat and thin types. The initial disease tends to become fat-hot type while the chronic disease tends to become thin-cold type. The cold type is treated with *Mùxiāngwán* (木香圓 *Costusroot Pill*) while the hot type is treated mainly with *Huángliánwán* (黃連圓 *Chinese Goldthread Pill*). The mixed cold-hot type is especially better to be treated with *Rúshèngwán* (如聖圓, *Saint-Like Pill*). After all, the young children's viscera are tender and weak and it is not allowed to attack drastically; drastic purgation will exhaust the liquid and fluid and lead to infantile malnutrition. For any case with indication of purgation, the severity as well as deficiency or excess should be differentiated and then the purgation can be given lest infantile malnutrition develops. At the initial stage, the liquid and fluid are decreased and the treatment should be to enrich liquid and fluid in the stomach mainly with *Báizhúsǎn* (白术散 *Powder of Rhizoma Atractylodis Macrocephalae*), which should be taken more in order to get better effect. The other conditions are seen in the following sections.

54

Disharmony of Stomach Qi

胃气不和

The child has lustless face, spiritless eyes, cold breath from the mouth, no appetite for food and vomiting water and the treatment should be to supplement spleen mainly with *Yìhuángsǎn* (益黄散 *Benefiting Yellow (Spleen) Powder*).

55

Cold and Deficient Stomach

胃冷虚

The child has lustless and pale face, thin and weak body, abdominal pain and no appetite for food, and the prescription should be to supplement spleen mainly with *Yìhuángsǎn* (益黃散 *Benefiting Yellow (Spleen) Powder*). If there is diarrhea, *Tiáozhōngyuán* (調中圓 *Middle-Regulating Pill*) is mainly applied.

56

Pain Due to Food Retention

积痛

The child has warm breath from the mouth, sallow and pale complexion, spiritless eyes or more white of the eyes, as well as drowsiness, fearing of eating or sour-smell stool; the treatment should be to resolve food retention with *Xiāojīyuán* (消積圓 *Resolving Food Retention Pill*). For the more severe case, *Báibǐngzǐ* (白餅子 *Medicinal White Muffin*) should be given for purgation and later for harmonizing stomach.

57

Pain Due to Worm Diseases

虫痛 (虚实腹痛附)

The child has lustless pale complexion, abdominal and heart pain, spitting spittle and plain water as well as pain at certain times, which is treated mainly with *Ānchóngsăn* (安蟲散 *Parasite-Expelling Powder*). Children have feeble constitution innately, so most of them suffer from this disease. There is pain due to retention, food or deficiency, which is the same in essentials while different in minor points. Only the child with pain due to parasite has tastelessness in the mouth with spittle flowing out spontaneously, which is treated according to the special manifestations.

58

Similarity Between Worms Syndrome and Epilepsy

虫与痫相似

The child has weak constitution innately, so there appears deficient cold of stomach to disturb parasite action and this causes heart pain. It is similar to epilepsy but there is no strabismus and hands spasm. This is treated mainly with *Ānchóngsăn* (安蟲散 *Parasite-Expelling Powder*).

59

Qi Disharmony

气不和

There is frequent puckering of lips and the Qi of spleen and stomach should be regulated mainly with *Yìhuángsǎn* (益黄散 *Benefiting Yellow (Spleen) Powder*).

60

Indigestion of Food

食不消

The child has cold spleen and stomach, so he cannot digest the food, and it should be treated by supplementing spleen, mainly with *Yìhuángsǎn* (益黄散 *Benefiting Yellow (Spleen) Powder*).

61

Aggregation in the Abdomen

腹中有癖

If the child has no appetite for food but can suck milk, it should be gradually purged *with Báibǐngzǐ* (白餅子 *Medicinal White Muffin*).

The child suffers from aggregation due to indigestion of milk and it tends to be incubated in the abdomen. There exist alternate chill and fever, drinking more water, panting or cough, which is similar to tidal fever and will progress to infantile malnutrition if not treated early. If there is aggregation in the abdomen, it will make the child have no appetite and result in deficient spleen and stomach with fever, so that the child feels thirst for water. With too much drinking, the water will wash down intestines and stomach, leading to loss of liquid and fluid. Spleen and stomach cannot transport and transform water and grain and the child has sunken and thin pulse as well as increasing anorexia. Deficiency of spleen and stomach causes inability to raise four limbs and subsequently evil will emerge; few children without being emaciated can progress to infantile malnutrition. Other prescriptions can be seen in the chapter of infantile malnutrition.

62

Deficient and Excessive Abdominal Distention and Swelling

虚实腹胀肿 (附)

Abdominal distention is due to deficiency of spleen and stomach as well as attack of disordered Qi. The excessive case has restlessness, distention and panting which can be purged with *Zǐshuāngyuán* (紫霜圓 *Purple Cream Pill*) and *Báibǐngzǐ* (白餅子 *Medicinal White Muffin*); if there is no panting, it is deficiency syndrome and it is not allowed to purge. If given purgation wrongly, it will cause deficiency of spleen Qi which spreads into lung, so that both lung and spleen (child-organ and mother-organ) are deficient. Lung governs the organs like eye balls and cheeks while spleen governs four limbs; if the mother-organ is deficient, there will be swelling of eye balls and cheeks. If there appears sallow complexion, it corresponds to spleen and is treated with *Tāqìwán* (塌氣圓 *Distention-Bleeded Pill*) for gradual effect; if not being cured, the number of pills can be increased but the drastic warm medicinals like *Dīngxiāng* (丁香 *los Syzygii Aromatici*), *Mùxiāng* (木香 *Radix Aristolochiae*), *Júpí* (橘皮 *Pericarpium Citri Reticulatae*),

80

Dòukòu (豆蔻 *Fructus Amomi Rotundus*), are not allowed. Why? If the deficient Qi of spleen hasn't emerged, and there is abdominal distention and no panting, the dispersing medicinals can be used in treatment, in order to disperse the deficient Qi in the upper and lower Jiao respectively; thus the disease can be cured. If the deficient Qi of spleen has emerged and spread into lung, it leads to internal deficiency of spleen and stomach; as soon as deficient Qi emerges, it will spread into four limbs, face and eyes (leading to swelling). Since the young child is susceptible to deficiency and excess and deficient spleen cannot tolerate cold and hot medicinals, taking the cold medicinals will cause cold syndrome while taking the hot medicinals will cause hot syndrome, and doctors cannot make mistakes in the treatment. Long-term deficient fever in stomach often leads to jaundice. Or the young child drinks too much water so that deficient spleen cannot dominate kidney; the deficient Qi will go upward and flow along four limbs, leading to edema; kidney water overflowing to lung results in gasping and it should be treated with *Tāqìyuán(wán)* (塌氣圓 *Distention-Bleeded Pill*). After being cured, there may still appear reddish complexion because the young child hasn't recovered from deficiency.

The treatment of abdominal distention is just like troops who are ordered to fight against enemy in the forest. When the enemies don't run away from the forest, a force can be concentrated to attack and win the battle; when the enemy have run away from the forest, the hurried attack is not allowed and otherwise the attack will fail; instead an effective tactic should be taken to catch the enemies gradually, which is the correct method.

In order to treat deficient abdominal distention, *Tāqìwán* (塌氣圓 *Distention-Bleeded Pill*) is first applied. If not cured, and there appear food retention, feces consolidation, dark yellowish urine, slight panting sometimes, hidden and excessive pulse, thirst for water sometimes and ability to eat, purgation is allowed. Because the spleen deficiency appears first and later there are food retention and feces consolidation, it is better to supplement spleen first and later to apply purgation; after purgation, supplementation of spleen is added again and the disease can be cured; supplementing lung wrongly is possible to cause deficient panting.

63

Frequent Sweating

喜汗

There is profuse sweating on the frontal head when the child wears thick clothes while sleeping, and it is treated mainly with *Zhǐhànsǎn* (止汗散 *Anti-Perspiration Powder*).

64

Night Sweats

盗汗

Night sweats are the occurrence of excessive sweating when sleeping due to deficiency of muscles and it is treated mainly with *Zhǐhànsǎn* (止汗散 *Anti-Perspiration Powder*). If there is sweating all over the body, it is treated mainly with *Xiāngguāyuán(wán)* (香瓜圓 *Fragrant Cucumber Pill*).

65

Night Crying

夜啼

The disease is due to cold spleen with abdominal pain and it should be treated with the medicinals of warming middle-Jiao as well as holding rite to exorcise evil; it is treated mainly with *Huāhuǒgāo* (花火膏 *Candlewick Powder*).

66

Crying Due to Fright

惊啼

When heat evil invades heart (mind), the treatment should be to tranquilize mind mainly with *Ānshényuán* (安神圓 *Mind-Tranquilizing Pill*).

67

Tongue Wagging

弄舌

Slightly hot spleen makes tongue collaterals slightly tight and the child frequently wags its tongue. In treatment, cold medicinals are not allowed for purgation and a small dosage of *Xièhuángsǎn* (瀉黃散 *Powder of Purging Yellow (Liver Fire)*) should be given gradually. There is also thirst for water, and the doctors suspect it is heat syndrome and give the cold medicinals for purgation, which is a wrong approach. In fact the cause of thirst for water is deficient heat of spleen and stomach leading to loss of liquid. If complicated by sallow complexion and thin body as well as vexing heat in five centers, it will progress to infantile malnutrition and it is better to apply *Húhuángliányuán* (胡黃連圓 *Pill of Rhizoma Picrorhizae*). If the serious illness hasn't been cured and there appears tongue wagging, the prognosis is very poor.

68

Erysipelas

丹瘤

When heat toxin invades the interstitial striae and struggles with blood-Qi, the evil emerges exteriorly and makes skin red like cinnabar, which should be treated with *Báiyùsăn* (白玉散 *White-Jade-like Powder*).

69

Open Fontanelles

解颅

The fontanelles are not closed due to deficiency of kidney Qi. After growing up, the child will have fewer smiles as well as more eye-white, lustless complexion, thin body and more anxiety and less joy. In addition the manifestations of kidney deficiency are seen.

70

Deficient Sweating of Taiyang Meridian

太阳虚汗

If there is sweating from the head to nape but not through the chest, it needn't be treated.

71

Sweating Due to Feeble Stomach Qi

胃怯汗

There is sweating from the head to the navel, which is associated with stomach deficiency, and it should be treated by supplementing stomach mainly with *Yìhuángsǎn* (益黄散 *Benefiting Yellow (Spleen) Powder*).

72

Crying Due to Stomach Deficiency

胃啼

Because the infantile sinews, bones and blood vessels have not developed fully, most infants tend to cry, which is the common phenomenon in infancy.

73

Neonatal Obesity

胎肥

After birth the newborn has thick muscles and ruddy skin all over the body; after one month the baby becomes thinner and thinner, has pinkish sclera, vexing heat in five centers, difficult defecation and frequent drooling, and it is treated mainly with *Yùtǐfǎ* (浴體法 *Medicinal Bath Therapy*).

74

Feeble Fetal Qi

胎怯

If the newborn has lustless complexion, thin muscles, whitish watery stool, no ruddy color of the body, frequent stuffiness, more retching and spiritless eyes, it should be treated with *Yùtǐfǎ* (浴體法 *Medicinal Bath Therapy*).

75

Fetal Heat

胎热

After birth the newborn has much blood-Qi, loud crying some-times, high body fever with skin having color like slight tea, reddish eyes, brownish urine, viscous stool and eagerness to suck milk; it should be treated with *Yùtǐfǎ* (浴體法 *Medicinal Bath Therapy*). The fatness or thinness of parents should be observed, and it is no good for fat parents to have a thin child, and vice versa.

76

Eagerness to Suck Milk in Vain

急欲乳不能食

Because the wind evil invades the navel of the infant and then flows into meridians of heart and spleen, the infant has thick tongue and dry lips so that the infant cannot suck milk, which should be treated by cooling heat evil from heart and spleen meridians.

77

Tortoise-Like Back and Chest

龟背龟胸

There is lung heat to cause bloating lung, which attacks chest and diaphragm leading to tortoise-like chest. Another cause is that the lactating woman prefers to have five kinds of spicy food. After birth, the wind evil invades the spine and damages the spinal cord, which can also cause the tortoise-like back. It is treated by putting drops of tortoise urine on the spinal vertebrae. The method to receive the urine of tortoise is as follows: put a tortoise on lotus leaf and then mirror it; the tortoise will pass urine spontaneously and finally its urine can be collected into a container.

78

Swelling Disease

肿病

When kidney heat spreads into bladder, it causes heat exuberance of bladder which then reversely goes to spleen and stomach; this is because spleen and stomach are too weak to restrain kidney (water) and kidney (water) retro-restrains (spleen) earth. Since spleen not only is associated with transportation and transformation of water but also governs four limbs, the water overflows all over the body to cause general and facial swelling. There is heavy panting with the severe condition. Why? Kidney is in great dominance to retro-restrain (spleen) earth; so in the upper region, kidney (water) restrains heart fire that restrains lung (metal); it leads to panting because lung is restrained by heart (fire). Maybe somebody will ask: "If heart (fire) punishes lung (metal), lung will manifest in deficiency; and now why is there excessive panting?" The answer is that there are two conditions: the first is heavy panting due to lung Qi surging because of reversal Qi of five solid viscera; the second is that Qi of kidney water overflows upward and invades lung, leading to heavy panting.

79

Mutual Dominance Among Five Solid Viscera and Their Severity of the Diseases

五脏相胜轻重

Liver diseases are often seen in autumn and liver is strong with exuberant wood (fire) which will retro-restrain lung (metal), so it is better to supplement lung and purge liver (fire). The mild case will subside while the severe case will die with white lips.

Lung diseases are often seen in spring and exuberant lung (metal) dominates liver, which should be treated by purging lung. The mild case will subside while the severe case will have bluish sclera of the eyes which must progress to fright. In addition, there is reddish sclera and the case must progress to convulsions; if it is due to feeble liver, there must be bluish sclera of the eyes.

Heart diseases are often seen in winter and heart fire is exuberant, which will retro-restrain kidney (water), so the treatment should be to supplement kidney (water) and subdue heart (fire). The mild case will subside while the severe case

99

will have inability to speak due to disease spreading down, which indicates feeble kidney Qi.

Kidney diseases are often seen in summer because water dominates fire, that is, kidney dominates heart, and kidney should be treated. The mild case will subside while the severe case will have palpitations and even convulsions.

Spleen diseases are often seen in the end of four seasons and are treated according to the rules mentioned above. The compliance is easy to treat while the reversal is difficult to treat. The child with feeble spleen will have reddish and sallow complexion and eyes. If the relationship among five solid viscera is disordered in reversal, the treatment is based on the syndromes concerned.

80

Miscellaneous Diseases

杂病症

Reddish and bluish eyes indicate approaching convulsions; staring eyes with bluish color and opisthotonus indicate convulsions; and severe stiff jaw indicates approaching seizure.

Spitting spittle from the mouth indicates pain later caused by worm diseases.

Drowsiness, frequent sneezing and palpitation indicate approaching pox and rash.

Vomiting, diarrhea, drowsiness and open eyes when sleeping indicate deficient fever of stomach; vomiting, diarrhea, drowsiness and not open eyes when sleeping indicate excessive heat of stomach. Vomiting, diarrhea and indigestion of milk indicate impaired digestion which is treated with purgation.

Vomiting spittle and sputum or whitish-greenish water indicates deficient cold of stomach; vomiting viscous drool and blood indicates lung heat; long-term lung heat will progress to deficiency.

Diarrhea with yellowish, reddish, deep reddish or blackish stool indicates heat syndrome and deep reddish stool indicates toxic heat. Diarrhea with bluish and whitish stool and indigestion of milk and grain indicate cold stomach.

Body fever without thirst for water indicates external heat while body fever with thirst for water indicates internal heat.

Lockjaw for a long time indicates dysphonia while it is also the case with delayed speech acquisition.

As a baby grows older, the toddler still cannot walk, and even if it can, its legs are weak. The teeth cannot erupt, and even if in eruption, the teeth are not firm. The infant has a very slow hair growth, and even the baby can grow out hair, it is not so glossy black.

Blood feeble deficiency is due to over-restraining by cold, leading to purplish lips.

Long-term brownish urine will lead to bloody urine. Long-term urinary stoppage will lead to full distention and it should be treated by promoting urination.

If the navel is not wiped dry after bath, the wind evil will invade through the navel to cause the sore and make the infant have closing mouth; the severe case is due to spleen deficiency.

Spitting hot spittle is treated with purgation therapy; spitting cold spittle is treated with warm therapy.

With pustule first and macule later, it is reversal syndrome; with pustule first and rash later, it is compliance syndrome; with blister first and rash later, it is reversal syndrome. With pustule first and blister later, mostly it belongs to compliance syndrome; with blister first and macule later, mostly it belongs to reversal syndrome. With rash first and macule later, it belongs to compliance syndrome. If there appears general pox and rash, it has good prognosis.

If the fetal Qi is substantial, there appear reddish complexion, more black of eyes and much joyful smile; if the fetal Qi is feeble, there appear sallow complexion, less black of eyes and more crying.

If the deficiency develops first or the previous purgation therapy is adopted in excess, it is better to supplement mother-organ first and later to purge it. If there is lung deficiency with excessive phlegm, it can be given purgation with the method of supplementing spleen first and purging lung later.

Sucking milk after great joy mostly leads to epileptic fright.

Sucking milk after wailing mostly leads to vomiting and diarrhea.

Heart pain with vomiting water is caused by the parasitic pain; heart pain without vomiting water is caused by cold heartache; vomiting water without heartache is caused by cold stomach.

The young child with the severe disease has five kinds of complexion, changeable and lustless, which indicates death.

Yawning with reddish complexion is due to wind heat; yawning with bluish complexion is due to frightened epilepsy; yawning with yellowish complexion is due to frightened epilepsy of spleen deficiency; yawing with drowsiness is due to internal heat; and yawning with hot breath is due to coryza.

After heat syndrome is treated with promoting urination or resolving toxic heat, there is no deficiency; warm supplementation is not allowed, otherwise the heat evil will recur.

81

Incurable Diseases

不治证

The red vessels in the eyes go through the pupil.
Bulging or sunken fontanelles.
Dry and black nose.
Dyspnea with fish-like mouth.
Vomiting worms incessantly.
Constant diarrhea with good spirit instead.
Great thirst and thirst recurring after temporary relief.
No sneezing after blowing medicinal powder into nose.
Severe disease, dry mouth and insomnia.
Affected by seasonal evil Qi and bluish and blackish spots on the lips.
Deep reddish cheeks as if applying rouge.
Nasal flaring.
Continuous dyspnea.

Part II
Medical Cases

Case 1

The assistant officer Li's son, at the age of three, suffered from convulsions from five-to-six to nine-to-ten in the morning. After several consultations, the disease hadn't been relieved and then Li called in Dr. Qian to inspect the child. Dr. Qian found that, when the child had convulsions, there was right strabismus and loud crying. Li asked: "Why does the baby have right strabismus during convulsions?" Qian answered: "It is a reversal syndrome." Li asked: "Why is it called a reversal?" Qi answered: "Male corresponds to Yang and nystagmus should have occurred in the left eye while female corresponds to Yin and nystagmus should have occurred in the right eye. When the boy's eyes are squinting to the left, he will not make any noise during attack and when squinting to the right, he will make a noise; when the girl's eyes are squinting to the right during attack, she will not make any noise, and when squinting to the left, she will make a noise. The mechanism is that, liver corresponds to the left while lung, to the right, and liver corresponds to wood while lung, to metal; if a male's eyes are squinting to the right, it means that lung dominates liver and metal punishes wood; if two solid viscera are struggling with each other, there will develop noise. The treatment principle is to purge exuberance and supplement weakness. The excessive evil of heart should be purged while it is not allowed to purge lung. With deficient lung there appear restlessness, choking and long exhalation; suffering from this disease, the male and female have contrast manifestations, so it is easier to treat male patient than female. If suffering from the attack, the female is squinting to the left; because lung dominates liver and the disease occurs in the autumn; as lung is in exuberance and liver cannot bear it, there appears crying. It should be prescribed to purge lung drastically, and later to purge heart fire and supplement liver. The reason that the patient has nystagmus and staring eyes is that liver governs eyes. Any convulsions are caused by wind and heat struggling with each other and wind pertaining to liver, so it is reflected in the eyes." Then Dr. Qian used *Xièfèitāng* (瀉肺湯 *Decoction of Purging Lung*) to purge it and after two days restlessness disappeared, showing that lung disease was subsiding. Later *Dìhuángyuán* (地黃圓 *Rehmaniae Pill*) was applied to enrich kidney and after three doses, *Xièqīngyuán* (瀉青圓 *Purging Blue (liver fire) pill*) and *Liángjīngyuán* (涼驚圓 *Fright-Cooling Pill*) were taken for two doses respectively. When medicinals to purge heart and liver were used, the disease could be cured in five days and the treatment could not be changed rashly. It was said that it was not allowed to purge deficient lung. Why? Dr. Qian answered: "If a male is squinting to the left, it is due to wood retro-restraining metal and exuberant liver dominating lung, and only liver needs to be purged. Alternately if the disease occurs in spring and summer when metal Qi is extremely deficient, lung should be supplemented and purgation should be avoided as caution."

Case 2

The seventh son of the royal living in Guangqin Palace, at the age of seven, had tidal fever for several days and was going to be cured. Dr. Qian told the child's father the Second King: "Your seventh son will recover from tidal fever but you should prevent the eighth son from convulsions." The king was angry and said: "You are only required to cure the disease of my seventh son and needn't say that my eighth son will have illness." However, Dr. Qian continued: "If your eighth son can get through tomorrow noon, he will have no suffering." As expected, the son suddenly had acute convulsions prior to that time. Dr. Qian was called in for treatment, and the son's disease was cured after three days. The key in the case was that, Dr. Qian found the eighth son of the king had staring eyes and reddish cheek and Qian considered it as heat syndrome of both liver and heart undoubtedly; moreover the son liked to sit on the stone stool for cooling, which reflected the extreme heat. The son had a fat physique including muscles and skin innately, with acute and rapid pulse, which indicated necessarily approaching convulsions. As to the time point of attack predicted, the heart and liver tend to take actions from 3–5 am to 11–13 at noon; after the treatment of purging heart and liver fire as well as nourishing kidney, the patient will be safe certainly.

Case 3

The grandson of Mr. Li, a financial officer, was at the age of 100 days and had an attack of convulsions for three to five times. Many doctors consulted treated the disease as infantile convulsions or epilepsy due to fetal fright but none of them had a positive response. Later Dr. Qian used *Dàqīnggāo* (大青膏 *Great Green Paste*) as much as a small bean with only one dose to disperse wind and heat. In addition, using the method of *Túxìnfǎ* (塗囟法 *Therapy of Applying Paste over Fontane*) and *Yùtǐfǎ* (浴體法 *Medicinal Bath Therapy*), the disease was cured in three days. Why did it have such a good effect? When wind invades the internal body and the infant cannot tolerate it, the infant will have an attack of convulsions. Frequent attacks indicate the mild disease. Why? Because the wind evil invades internally, and whenever the child cannot tolerate it, the convulsions will occur. If there appear sparse attacks, it indicates that the disease originates from the internal viscera and cannot be rescued. With frequent attacks, it is suitable to disperse wind and cold with *Dàqīnggāo* (大青膏 *Great Green Paste*). The medicine is not allowed to take too much, because the infant is too young and susceptible to deficiency and excess; taking too much will lead to heat; only one dose is enough and with additional therapies of *Yùtǐfǎ* (浴體法 *Medicinal Bath Therapy*), few cases are ineffective.

Case 4

In the East Capital, the son of Mr. Wang had vomiting and diarrhea, and many doctors consulted treated it with purgative thearpy, which caused extreme deficiency, and the disease turned into chronic convulsions. Its clinical manifestations included opening eyes when sleeping, spasm of hands and feet as well as cold body. Dr. Qian said: "This is chronic infantile convulsions which can be treated with *Guālóutāng* (蔴藪湯 *Trichosanthis Decoction*)." Because the baby had full stomach Qi, he could open eyes when sleeping with warm body after medication. Moreover Mr. Wang suspected his son couldn't excrete and called in doctors. They treated it with purgative therapy and prescribed *Bāzhèngsǎn* (八正散 *Eight-Ingredient-Rectificating Powder*) and the like and after several doses the child still had no excretion and there appeared cold body again. Dr. Qian was consulted for urination, but Dr. Qian said that it was not suitable to promote urination and otherwise it would lead to cold body. Mr. Wang said: "The body has been cold," and then held the baby out. Dr. Qian said: "The baby cannot eat leading to deficiency in stomach, and with promoting excretion, the baby will die. A long-term deficiency of spleen and kidney will lead to cold body and opening eyes when sleeping. Fortunately, the fetal Qi is full which is difficult to be worn away." Dr. Qian applied *Yihuángsǎn* (益黄散

Benefiting Yellow (Spleen) Powder) and *Shǐjūnzǐyuán* (使君子圓
Fructus Quisqualis Pill) for four doses and let the baby eat a
little food. By noon, he was able to eat as expected. The mechanism is that promoting excretion will lead to deficiency of
spleen and stomach and it should be prescribed to supplement
spleen and avoid purgation. Later the child was found unable
to speak and many doctors treated it as aphonia. Dr. Qian said:
"Since it is aphonic, why can the baby open his eyes and eat?
And why can the baby have neither tight mouth nor trismus."
Some doctors did not know the mechanism. Instead, Dr. Qian
applied *Dìhuángyuán* (地黃圓 *Rehmaniae Pill*) to nourish kidney. The mechanism was that using clearing medicinals to
promote urination led to both deficiency of spleen and kidney.
Now spleen Qi had been full but kidney was still deficient, so
nourishing kidney could relieve the disease. After half a month
of treatment, the baby could speak and after one month the
disease was cured.

Case 5

Mr. Du was the owner of a TCM pharmacy in the East Capital. He had a son at the age of five who suffered from cough from the 11th lunar month in the previous year to the third lunar month in the current year and the cough hadn't been relieved. At the onset the child had cough with spitting and it was affected by external wind and cold which accumulated in the lung meridian, leading to lung disease. The cough and spitting indicated the wind evil in lung. It was suitable to use *Máhuáng* (麻黃 *Herba Ephedrae Sinicae*) and the like for dispersion and later to use cooling medicinals to clear internal heat and the cough could be cured. However, at that time some doctors used *Tiěfěnwán* (鐵粉圓 *Iron-powder Pill*), *Bànxiàyuán* (半夏圓 *Pill of Rhizoma Pinelliae*) and *Biǎnyínwán* (褊銀圓 *Flat Mercury Pill*) for purgation which caused lung deficiency and worsening cough; till the first three months of spring the disease hadn't been cured. Dr. Qian was consulted for inspection and the child's manifestations included bluish complexion with some luster, cough with panting, choking sometimes with long exhalation. Dr. Qian said: "The body is encumbered with phlegm and damp with a ratio of eight-nine in ten. The mechanism is that the child has bluish complexion with some luster, indicating the exuberance of liver Qi. The three months of spring is the period that liver acts and lung declines. Cough is

113

the symptom of lung disease. The child's lung disease lingers from the 11th lunar month previous year to the third lunar month this year and the long-term disease leads to deficiency and withering of lung. After the child was given purgation and because spleen and lung have the relation of child- and mother-organ and both spleen and lung are dominated by liver, the reversal syndrome developed. So the child had cough with panting, choking and long exhalation." Dr. Qian urgently gave *Xièqīngyuán* (瀉青圓 *Purging Blue Pill*) for purgation and later *Ejiāosǎn* (阿膠散 *Donkey-Hide Gelatin Powder*) for supplementation of lung. Next day the child still had bluish complexion but no luster. Dr. Qian again applied supplementation of lung but the child coughed as before. Additionally Dr. Qian applied purgation of liver, but before the completion of purging liver, the disease was complicated by lung deficiency with pale lips like white silk. Dr. Qian said: "The child with the disease is doomed to die, which is incurable. Why? Because liver is drastically exuberant while lung is critically deficient; the lung disease occurs at an improper time, so liver dominates it. Now I applied purgation of liver for three times but the lung disease still doesn't subside, and supplementation of lung also for three times but lung deficiency still exists; the child will not live long, that is, the prognosis will be death. If the disease occurs in autumn, the child can be rescued with a probability of three-four in ten. But if it occurs in spring and summer, it is difficult to be cured by one in ten." As expected the child finally died with drastic panting.

Case 6

Mr. Li, a transportation officer in Jingdong (Now South of Shangqiu City in Henan Province), had a grandson at the age of eight years old who suffered from couging, chest fullness and shortness of breath. The doctor said that there was heat evil in the lung meridian and gave *Zhúyètāng* (竹葉湯 *Decoction of Olium Phyllostachytis Henonis*) and *Niúhuánggāo* (牛黄膏 *Calculus Bovis Paste*) for two doses respectively in the treatment; after three days the panting became worse. Dr. Qian said: "It is due to deficiency of lung Qi complicated by cold evil, leading to panting and chest fullness. It should be given invigoration of lung and avoid cooling medicinals." Mr. Li said: "The doctor has applied *Zhúyètāng* (竹葉湯 *Decoction of Olium Phyllostachytis Henonis*) and *Niúhuánggǎo* (牛黄膏 *Calculus Bovis Paste*)." Dr. Qian asked the doctor: "Why did you treat in this way?" The doctor answered: "In order to reduce fever and decrease drooling." Dr. Qian asked: "Where does the heat come from?" The doctor answered: "The heat lingering in the lung meridian causes cough and a long-term cough without relief causes drooling." Qian Yi said: "The child is deficient innately and affected by wind and cold, and where does the heat evil come from? If it were treated as lung heat,

115

why don't you treat lung instead of regulating heart? Both *Zhúyètāng* (竹葉湯 *Decoction of Olium Phyllostachytis Henonis*) and *Niúhuánggǎo* (牛黃膏 *Calculus Bovis Paste*) are applied to treat heart heat." The doctor felt ashamed and later Dr. Qian cured the case.

Case 7

Mr. Zhang, living in the East Capital, had a grandson at the age of nine years old, who suffered from lung fever. Some doctors treated it with *Shèxiāng* (麝 *Moschus*), *Shēngxījiǎo* (犀 *Cornu Rhinoceri Asiatici*), *Niúhuáng* (生牛黄 *Calculus Bovis*), *Zhēnzhū* (珠 *Margarita*) and *Lóngnǎo* (龍 *Borneolum Syntheticum*); after one month the illness hadn't been cured. The manifestations included cough, panting, chest tightness, restlessness, constant thirst for water, and complete anorexia. Dr. Qian applied *Shǐjūnzǐyuán* (使君子圓 *Fructus Quisqualis Pill*) and *Yìhuángsǎn* (益黄散 *Benefiting Yellow (Spleen) Powder*). Mr. Zhang asked: "The child has heat originally and why do you again apply warm medicinals?" Other doctors used cooling medicinals for purgation but after one month the therapy was ineffective. Dr. Qian said: "Long-term cooling medication leads to cold and anorexia, and the young child has deficiency with anorexia which should be given to supplement spleen. When the child restores the normal diet, lung meridian can be purged and the disease must be cured." After taking medication for invigorating lung for two days, Mr. Zhang's grandson can eat; and then Dr. Qian gave *Xièbáisǎn* (瀉白散 *Purging*

White Powder) to purge lung heat and the disease was cured completely. Mr. Zhang asked: "Why does the child have no deficiency after the therapy?" Dr. Qian answered: "First to invigorate spleen and later to purge lung heat, so there appears no deficiency."

Case 8

The king in Muqin Palace had the tenth son, who suffered from pox and rash, and many doctors were consulted for treatment. The king asked: "The rash hasn't erupted and what organ does it relate to?" One doctor said it was the syndrome of drastic heat, one doctor said that it was the lingering of cold-damage, and another doctor said there was some toxin in the womb of the pregnant mother. Dr. Qian said: "If it is related to stomach heat, why does the child have alternative chill and heat? If there is some toxin in the womb of the pregnant mother, what organ is it related to?" The doctor replied: "To the spleen and stomach." Dr. Qian said: "Since the focus is in spleen and stomach, why does the child have fright-convulsions?" The doctor had nothing to reply. Dr. Qian said: "When the fetus is in the womb, the human body is formed in the sixth or seventh month and it is possible for the fetus to absorb the turbid liquid into five viscera from the mother. Till the tenth month, the turbid liquid fills the stomach. At birth there is something dirty in the mouth, and there will be no illness as long as the mother wipes the baby's mouth clean with her hands. In folk medicine the juice of *Huánglián* (黄連 *Rhizoma Coptidis*) is used to purge the meconium and dirty phlegm. These is also the turbid factor from the mother when the residual Qi of the toxin in the womb spreads into the viscera of fetus, and obviously the disease is caused by the previous factor complicated by invasion of slight cold into the body. When pox and rash haven't erupted, the manifestations corresponding to five solid viscera can be found, and if some solid viscera is more affected by the turbid factor, there will develop pox and rash. At the onset, the baby tends to have yawning first, sudden stuffiness, fright-convulsion, alternate chill and fever, cold hands and feet, dried red face and cheeks, cough and sometimes sneezing, all of which are corresponding symptoms of five solid viscera respectively. Yawning and stuffiness are associated with liver, sometimes fright-convulsion is associated with heart; alternate chill and fever as well as cold hands and feet are associated with spleen; red face and cheeks as well as cough are associated with lung; only kidney has no according manifestations because kidney is located below and has no chance to absorb the turbid liquid. Any fetal pox and rash are the toxic reflection of five solid viscera. If classified by eruptive features, blister involves liver, pustule involves lung, macula involves heart and rash involves spleen; only kidney doesn't absorb turbid toxin and has no according signs. However the black pox is associated with kidney as it was carelessly affected by wind and cold as well as hunger, which is due to internal deficiency." Also *Bàolóngyuán* (抱龍圓 *Holding Dragon Pill*) was given for several doses and finally the disease was cured without any other manifestations. If pox and rash haven't erupted, the specific manifestations according to five solid viscera respectively can be found; for the developed eruption, the pox and rash can be categorized to some solid viscus.

Case 9

The fifth son in the fourth King's palace suffered from fright-convulsions due to falling when playing on the swings; a doctor used heating medicinals but the disease was not cured after treatment.

Dr. Qian said: "The disease originally belongs to acute convulsions and later there is drastic heat in the body; it should be given antipyretic agents first." Then *Dàhuángyuán* (大黄圓 *Rhubarb Pill*), *Yùlùsǎn* (玉露散 *Jade Dew Powder*) and *Xīngxīngwán* (惺惺丸 *Alerting Pill*) are applied plus *Niúhuáng* (生牛黄 *Calculus Bovis*), *Lóngnǎo* (龍脑 *Borneolum Syntheticum*) and *Shèxiāng* (麝香 *Moschus*) to reduce fever in vain. On the third day of the course there appeared fever especially on the skin and muscles. Dr. Qian said: "If in two more days the disease is not cured, there must develop macula and sore, because the heat cannot be dispersed." The other doctor initially used dispersing agents to force heat evil into the exterior of the body and then there developed macula because of exterior heat. At the onset of acute fright-convulsion, doctors should have given the agents of relieving convulsions for purgation; now the application of dispersing agents was a reversal of treatment principle. Two days lager the maculae expectedly erupted. *Bìshènggāo* (必胜膏 *Succeeding Paste*) was applied in the treatment and seven days later the disease was cured.

Case 10

The first son of the prince in Muqin Palace suffered from pox and rash. Initially a doctor with surname Li was consulted, and later Dr. Qian was called in and he left three doses of *Bàolóngyuán* (抱龍圓 *Holding Dragon Pill*). Dr. Li used some medicinals for purgation but the rash became denser; Dr. Qian was startled upon inspection and said: "If purgative medicinals were not given, how could the case progress to the reversal syndrome?" The prince said: "Dr. Li has used some medicinals for purgation." Qian Yi said: "The rash begins to appear but there are not any other manifestations, so it is not allowed to apply purgative therapy. It is enough to use moderate medicine, increase times of milk-feeding and avoid wind-cold. If the rash does not come out in three days, or it does not come out rapidly, only a few agents to promote eruption are needed; if having no adequate eruption after slight medication, it is necessary to add medicinals; if no eruption, it is necessary to use drastic medications; if not much eruption after drastic medication with normal pulse and without any other signs, it indicates the rash is sparse originally and it is not allowed to promote eruption. With more excessive heat evil, it is necessary to promote urination; with slight heat evil, it is necessary to resolve the toxin; with rapid spreading, neither eruptive nor purgative therapy is allowed and only *Bàolóngyuán* (抱龍圓

Holding Dragon Pill) is applied for the treatment. When the rashes form scabs and the child can eat, do not withdraw *Dàhuáng yuán* (大黄圓 *Rhubarb Pill*) until the patient has diarrhea for one or two times. However purging therapy has been applied for one day but rashes fail to erupt completely with denser lesions; it indicates the refractory disease due to misuse of purgation. Even if the child can be out of danger, there are still three complications: presence of scabies, carbuncle and red eyes." Doctor Li failed to cure the disease, and after three days the rashes became black and sunken; Dr. Qian was called in again and said: "Fortunately there is no chill, indicating the disease hasn't been encumbered by a crisis." Therefore, *Bǎixiángyuán* (百祥圓 *Hundred Lucks Pill*) was applied with the aid of *Niúhuánggāo* (牛黄膏 *Calculus Bovis Paste*) in the treatment, one big dose respectively; till the fifth day the rashes were restored to red and vivid status and after seven days the rashes were cured. When the pox and rash become black, it indicates the disease has regressed to kidney; because kidney water is in exuberance which can reversely restrain spleen (earth) and earth cannot restrain water, leading to rigor due to spleen deficiency; so it is difficult to cure the disease. *Bǎixiángwán* (百祥圓 *Hundred Lucks Pill*) was used in order to purge the damp-heat in the bladder; if the bladder had no excessive evil, kidney naturally had no exuberance. Why not purge kidneys directly? Dr. Qian answered: "Because kidney is often in a deficient status, it cannot withstand the purgation. If the two doses of medication are still ineffective, the child will die due to complication of cold syndrome."

Case 11

Mr. Xu in the capital had a son, aged three, who suffered from tidal fever, with manifestations including convulsions when the sun was setting in the west, slight body fever, a little squint, opening eyes when sleeping, cold limbs, panting and yellowish stool. Then both Dr. Li and Dr. Qian were consulted for treatment. Dr. Qian asked Dr. Li: "Why does the child have convulsions?" Dr. Li answered: "Due to wind evil." Dr. Qian asked: "Why does the child have slight body fever?" Dr. Li answered: "Due to limbs twitching". Dr. Qian asked: "Why does the child have strabismus and opening eyes when sleeping?" Dr. Li answered: "The convulsions cause strabismus." Dr. Qian asked: "Why does the child have cold limbs?" Dr. Li answered: "Critically cold limbs must be caused by internal heat." Dr. Qian asked: "Why does the child have panting?" Dr. Li answered: "Because of the severe convulsions." Dr. Qian asked: "How do you treat the disease?" Dr. Li answered: "*Tìjīngyuán* (嚏驚圓 *Sneezing Pill for Reliving Convulsion*) can be delivered via the nostrils and convulsions must stop." Dr. Qian asked: "Since there is so-called wind-disease with slight body fever, strabismus and opening eyes when sleeping due to convulsions, cold limbs due to internal heat and panting due to more severe convulsions, what medicine are you going to apply for the treatment?" Dr. Li answered: "All of them can be treated with the same medicine." Dr. Qian said: "I don't think so. Uncontrolled muscle movement is associated with excessive liver Qi, leading to the convulsions; there appears slight body fever when the sun is setting to the west during which lung is taking action in its due time; because lung governs the body, the warm body with fever indicates lung deficiency. There is slight strabismus and opening eyes when sleeping because of liver (wood) retro-restraining lung (metal). Cold limbs are caused by spleen deficiency; If lung is seriously deficient, its mother-organ spleen is also deficient; thus wood Qi over-restrains spleen, leading to cold limbs. It should be firstly treated with *Yìhuángsǎn* (益黄散 *Benefiting Yellow (Spleen) Powder*) and *Ejiāosǎn* (阿膠散 *Donkey-Hide Gelatin Powder*); after lung deficiency subsides, it is later treated with *Xièqīngyuán* (瀉青圓 *Purging Blue (liver fire) pill*), *Dǎochìsǎn* (導赤散 *Purging Red* Powder) and *Liángjīngyuán* (涼驚圓 *Fright-Cooling Pill*)." The disease was cured after nine days.

Case 12

The son of Jianbu (equivalent to secretary at present) Zhu was five years old and had fever at night and the temperature returned to normal the next morning. Among many doctors consulted, some treated it as cold-damage and some treated it as heat disease with cooling medicinals to reduce fever in vain. The manifestations included much drool and drowsiness; other doctors applied *Tiěfěnwán* (鐵粉圓 *Iron-powder Pill*) to remove drool but the disease was worsening. On the fifth day, the child drank a lot of water because of thirst. Dr. Qian said: "It is not allowed to adopt purgation." Then *Báizhúsǎn* (白术散 *Powder of Rhizoma Atractylodis Macrocephalae*) *1 liang* (30 g) was used and decocted into three liters of medicinal liquid, so that the child could drink as much as possible at any time. Mr. Zhu asked: "Will it cause diarrhea to drink so much?" Dr. Qian replied: "If the child does not drink unboiled water, it is impossible to cause diarrhea, and even if having diarrhea, it's no surprise but what's more important is not to adopt purgation." Mr. Zhu asked: "What disease are you going to treat first?" Dr. Qian replied: "To relieve thirst and to resolve phlegm as well as to reduce fever and to clear the mind; all of these depend on this medicine." Till the evening all the medicinal liquid was finished; after checking, Dr. Qina said: "The child can have three more liters of medicinal liquid." And then *Báizhúsǎn* (白术散

Powder of Rhizoma Atractylodis Macrocephalae) was decocted to produce three more liters; after the child drank up the medicine, the disease began to subside. On the third day, the child drank three more liters of *Báizhúsǎn* (白术散 *Powder of Rhizoma Atractylodis Macrocephalae*) dedoction, and had no thirst and drooling. Later *Ājiāosǎn* (阿膠散 *Donkey-Hide Gelatin Powder*) was added, and after two doses, the disease was cured.

Case 13

Jianbu Zhu had a son at the age of three who suddenly developed a fever. Some doctors said: "It is the disease of heart heat." The evidence included red cheeks and lips, irritability and thirst for water; and then three doses of *Niúhuánggāo* (牛黄膏 *Calculus Bovis Paste*) were applied and the child took it with *Xièxīntāng* (瀉心湯 *Decoction of Purging Heart Fire*). The next day the disease was not improved and instead the child felt a malaise and had no appetite; then the purgative therapy was applied again and resultantly the child had diarrhea with yellow foaming stool. Dr. Qian said: "Now the heart meridian is deficient where the heat is lingering, and it is the cooling medicinals for purgation that cause the disease of deficient consumption." Dr. Qian first applied *Báizhúsǎn* (白术散 *Powder of Rhizoma Atractylodis Macrocephalae*) to generate the liquid in stomach and later *Shēngxīsǎn* (生犀散 *Powder of Raw rhinoceros horn*) to treat the underlined disease. Mr. Zhu asked: "How about treating the yellow foaming stool?" Dr. Qian replied: "As long as stomach Qi restores to the normal, diarrhea will stop spontaneously because it is a deficient fever." Zhu asked: "How about the application of *Xièxīntāng* (瀉心湯 *Decoction of Purging Heart Fire*)?" Dr. Qian replied: "Among the ingredients of *Xièxīntāng* (瀉心湯 *Decoction of*

Purging Heart Fire), *Huánglián* (黄連 *Rhizoma Coptidis*) is cold in nature; if the child takes it too much, it will cause diarrhea because of cooling spleen and stomach." After Dr. Qina Yi sat for a long time, many other doctors came to the Zhu family and said: "It is excessive fever indeed." Dr. Qian said: "It is deficient fever. If it were excessive fever, why did the child develop irritability, plus sallow complexion, red cheeks, vexing heat in five centers and no appetite with thirst for water?" Other doctors retorted: "Since it is deficient fever, why did the child have yellow foaming stool?" Dr. Qian smiled and said: "Yellow foaming stool reflects over medication of *Xièxīntāng* (瀉心湯 *Decoction of Purging Heart Fire*)." Later Dr. Qian gave *Húhuánglián yuán* (胡黄連圓 *Figwortflower Picrorhiza Rhizome Pill*) and the disease was cured.

Case 14

Mr. Zhang had three sons and all of his sons fell ill (one day): The eldest son sweated all over the body, the second son sweated from the vertex to the chest and the youngest had beads of sweat on his forehead. Some doctors treated the sweating with *Màijiānsǎn* (麥煎散 *Powder Decocted with Wheat*) in vain. Dr. Qian ordered: "The eldest is given *Xiāngguāyuán* (香瓜圓 *Pill of Fructus Cucumis Sativi*), the second is given *Yìhuángsǎn* (益黃散*Benefiting Yellow (Spleen) Powder*) and the youngest is given *Shígāotāng* (石膏湯 *Decoction of Gypsum Fibrosum*)." After five days, the three sons recovered from the illness.

Case 15

The fifth son of the fourth King in Guangqin Palace suffered from constant vomiting and diarrhea with undigested food; many doctors prescribed tonics and ordered them to be taken with ginger juice. In the sixth lunar month the child took the warm medicine for only one day and developed panting additionally and constant vomiting. Dr. Qian said: "The child should be given cooling medicinals for the treatment. The reason is that there is damage due to heat evil in the internal. Three doses of *Shígāotāng* (石膏湯 *Decoction of Gypsum Fibrosum*) can be taken at a time." Other doctors said: "For much vomiting and diarrhea with indigestion of food, spleen should be supplemented, and why do you use cooling medicinals?" The king believed in the words of other doctors and gave three doses of *Dīngxiāngsǎn* (丁香散 *Clove Flower Powder*). Later on Dr. Qian arrived and said: "It is not allowed to take this medicine and otherwise there will develop abdominal distension, body fever, thirst for water, vomiting and hiccups in three days." Three days later, everything was going as Dr. Qian expected. The reason for this is that, the weather is extremely hot in the sixth lunar month and it is easy for heat evil to invade the abdomen, leading to thirst for water; the heat evil damages spleen and stomach, leading to severe vomiting and diarrhea. However, some doctors again misused the warm

131

medicinals, so that there is also heat evil in upper-Jiao leading to panting and thirst for water; in this way the patient will die in three days. As other doctors failed to treat the disease, the king asked for Dr. Qian again to enter the Palace. Finding that the child had heat syndrome, Dr. Qian applied three doses of *Báihǔtāng* (白虎湯 *White Tiger Decoction*) together with *Báibǐngzi* (白餅子 *Medicinal White Muffin*) for purgation. After one day, the medicinal dosage was reduced by two in ten; on the second and third days, two more doses of *Báihǔtāng* (白虎湯 *White Tiger Decoction*) were given respectively; on the fourth day one dose of *Shígāotāng* (石膏湯 *Decoction of Gypsum Fibrosum*) was given again; and immediately, five pills made of *Màidōng* (麥門冬 *Radix Ophiopogonis Japonici*), *Huángqín* (黃芩 *Radix Scutellariae Baicalensis*), *Lóngnǎo* (腦子 *Borneolum Syntheticum*), *Niúhuáng* (牛黃 *Calculus Bovis*), *Tiānzhúhuáng* (天竺黃 *Concretio Silicea Bambusae*) and *Báifúlíng* (茯苓 *Poria*), coated with *Zhūshā* (砂 *Cinnabaris*) were taken with *Zhúyètāng* (竹葉湯 *Decoction of Olium Phyllostachytis Henonis*); in the end the fever was lowered down to the normal range and the child's health was restored.

Case 16

Mr. Feng was an assistant officer and had a son at the age of five who suffered from vomiting, diarrhea, high fever and anorexia. After inspection, Dr. Qian said: "The black color is less than the white in the child's eyes and there is pale complexion, indicating deficient spirit. The less black of eyes indicates kidney deficiency. The black of the eyes corresponds to kidney water; the sign can reflect the insufficient constitution and kidney deficiency, so the child is susceptible to illness. Even when the child grows up, he won't have firm skin and muscles and cannot tolerate freezing winter and hot summer; the child is prone to the deficient or excessive conditions, and his spleen and stomach are also deficient. In addition, he cannot indulge in drinking and sexual life; if he does not pay attention to maintenance, he cannot survive the middle age. The patient often has no spiritual and lustrous complexion, and his face is just like the face of a woman having menstrual bleeding. Now the child has vomiting, diarrhea, anorexia and high fever, due to maldigestion, and it is not allowed to give purgation, otherwise it will cause deficiency. The evil involving lung will cause cough; involving heart, palpitation; involving spleen, diarrhea; and involving kidney, more deficiency. It can be treated only with *Xiāojīyuán* (消積圓 *Resolving Food Retention*

Pill) for digestion, because it is only mild food retention. If it is a severe damage by improper diet, purgation can be adopted, and otherwise it will progress to aggregation. As long as there is excessive food retention internally, purgation can then be adopted. After purgation, supplementation must be adopted and the disease must be cured. The treatment varies depending on whether it is a deficient or excessive condition and would not be ineffective."

Case 17

The seventh son living in Guangqin King Palace was seven years old and suffered from vomiting and diarrhea during the lunar month of July. The clinical manifestations of the patient included complete anorexia, drowsiness, restlessness when sleeping, choking, retching with or without feces and no thirst. Many doctors treated it as fright and the fright was suspected of causing the drowsiness. Dr. Qian said: "The treatment should be first to supplement spleen, and later to reduce fever." Then *Shǐjūnzǐyuán* (使君子圓 *Fructus Quisqualis Pill*) was applied to supplement spleen and *Shígāotāng* (石膏湯 *Decoction of Gypsum Fibrosum*) to reduce fever. The next day both *Shuǐyín* (水银 *Hydrargyrum*) and *Liúhuáng* (硫磺 *Sulfur*) of *1* zi (0.45 g) were mixed with *Shēngjiāng* (生薑 *Rhizoma Zingiberis*) to take for purging the stagnation. Dr. Qian explained: "For any vomiting and diarrhea within five months, purgation is adopted by nine in ten and supplementation by one in ten. Within eight months, supplementation is given by ten in ten without purgation. This disease is diarrhea due to spleen deficiency but many doctors treated it wrongly, leading to deficient damage, and the application of purgation will cause death immediately. The spleen should be supplemented immediately, so the application of *Shǐjūnzǐyuán* (使君子圓 *Fructus Quisqualis Pill*) can improve the condition at once."

Dr. Qian also left the medicinals of warming stomach and benefiting spleen to stop the diarrhea. Dr. Li, a medical student, asked: "Why is the child retching after meal?" Dr. Qian replied: "The child has anorexia due to deficient spleen and less liquid causes retching." Li asked again: "Why does the child have greenish-brownish watery stool?" Dr. Qian replied: "Extremely deficient intestine and stomach will result in extreme cold." Resultantly the disease was cured by Dr. Qian's treatment.

Case 18

Mr. Huang, an assistant officer, had a son at the age of two, who suffered from diarrhea. Many doctors had applied the method of stopping diarrhea for ten days, and the manifestations included bluish and whitish watery stool with undigested milk food, cold body, choking and drowsiness. The doctors thought it as a critical disease. Dr. Qian Yi first applied three doses of *Yìhuángsǎn* (益黄散 Benefiting Yellow (Spleen) Powder) and three does of *Bǔfèisǎn* (補肺散 *Lung-Invigorating Powder*). Three days later, the child's body became warm and the choking disappeared, and then *Báibǐngzǐ* (白餅子 *Medicinal White Muffin*) was applied for mild purgation, together with two doses of *Yìpísǎn* (益脾散 *Spleen-invigorating Powder*), and the diarrhea was cured. Why was there such curative effect? This is because the diarrhea was originally caused by spleen deficiency due to damage of maldigestion; initially the patient was not given drastic purgation and the disease was delayed for ten days, so that there was excess in the upper region and deficiency in the lower region, weak spleen Qi and also lung deficiency. Therefore, after supplementation of spleen and lung, the disease was relieved, that is, the body became warm and choking disappeared. Some doctor asked:

"If the disease was caused by maldigestion, generally it is treated with purgation. Why don't you adopt purgation first and later supplementation?" Qian Yi replied: "The bluish stool indicates cold spleen; and if purgative therapy is applied first, it will cause drastic deficiency; so initially spleen and lung should be invigorated and later purgative therapy is applied, in order to avoid deficiency; after that supplementation is applied again."

Case 19

Mr. Wang, the king's son-in-law, had a son at the age of five, who had straightly staring eyes and was eating nothing. Some people said that it was caused by ghosts, so a witch was invited to burn ghost paper money for godliness; but the patient did not get better. Then Dr. Qian was consulted and Dr. Qian said: "This is the disease of internal visceral disorder, and why shall we bother ourselves by praying to god?" Dr. Qian gave *Xiègānyuán* (瀉肝圓 *Liver-purging Pill*) and the child's disease was cured.

Case 20

A woman with surname Xin had a daughter at the age of five who suffered from the disease of abdominal pain due to worms. Some doctors treated it with *Bādòu* (巴豆 *Fructus Crotonis*), *Gānqī* (乾漆 *ResinaToxicodendri*) and *Náoshā* (硇砂 *Sal Ammoniac*) in vain. On the fifth day of the course, the child developed frequent crying, restless sleeping in supine position, pressing the heart and abdomen regions herself, sometimes shouting, no normal complexion such as abnormal greenish, yellowish, blackish or whitish color, spiritless and dull eyes and white lips with spittle. On the sixth day, the child developed bloating chest and restless sleeping, and Dr. Qian was consulted. After careful inspection, Dr. Qian gave three doses of *Wúyísǎn* (蕪荑散 *Powder of Pasta Ulmi*); and later Dr. Qian was startled to find the child's eyeballs still with bluish color and said: "It is an extremely dangerous disease; if it is complicated by diarrhea, it will progress to a reversal syndrome." The next day, Xin met Dr. Qian and said: "On the third night watch the child had diarrhea." Dr. Qian looked at the feces which were like medicinal juice in the bedpan, and stirred them with a wooden stick and found some pills in the feces. Dr. Qian said: "The child has thick muscles indicating full Qi but now the child instead manifests deficiency, which is incurable." Ms. Xin asked: "Why is that so?" Dr. Qian replied: "The cold spleen and stomach cause disturbance of worms; now the child's eyeballs show a bluish color instead, indicating that liver over-restrains spleen, and complication by diarrhea indicates extremely deficient Qi. And pills are excreted with feces, reflecting Qi collapse of spleen and stomach; further there is uncooperative relation between physique and disease, so I know it is fatal." Five days later, the child became unconscious and died on the seventh day.

Case 21

Mr. Duan, a master of ceremonies, had a son at the age of four who suffered from cough, body fever, vomiting and much spittle, and after several days the child developed hemoptysis. The doctors consulted earlier treated with *Júgěngtāng* (桔梗湯 *Decoction of Radix Platycodonis*) and *Fángjǐyuán* (防己圓 *Pill of Radix StephaniaeTetrandrae*) in vain. The phlegm was surging upwards to cause constant vomiting and panting, and Dr. Qian was consulted. Dr. Qian gave a big dose of *Biǎnyínyuán* (褊銀圓 *Flat Mercury Pill*), together with *Bǔfèisǎn* (補肺散 *Lung-Invigorating Powder*) and *Bǔpísǎn* (補脾散 *Spleen-Invigorating Powder*) in the treatment. Some doctors asked: "Mr. Duan's son has hemoptysis due to lung deficiency, and why do you still adopt the purgative therapy?" Dr. Qian replied: "There is expectoration of blood from the lungs and it is due to heat evil; and the long-term disease will cause deficiency and withering of lungs. Now the phlegm is surging upwards to cause vomiting, so it should be given purgation to remove the phlegm. If there is no spittle surging upwards to cause vomiting, it is convenient to be treated, because vomiting and spittle can cause deficiency and also fright. The excessive phlegm surging upwards can also cause convulsions;

according to the treatment principle it is better to purge phlegm first and later to invigorate spleen and lung; as long as the spitting is stopped, vomiting can be cured, which is a compliant therapy. If you first invigorate lung, it is a reversal therapy. This is called treatment according to the severity and priority of the disease."

Case 22

Langzhong (equivalent to the director of bureau) Qi lived in Zheng country and his family liked to collect medicines for donation. His son suddenly suffered from visceral fever; Mr. Qi took out *Qīngjīngāo* (青金膏 *Blue-Golden Paste*) by himself and let the child take three doses as one big dose at one time. From the time of medication to the third night watch, the child had diarrhea for five times and developed drowsiness. Mr. Qi considered that the child had drowsiness due to fright. Then Mr. Qi gave his child another dose of *Qīngjīngāo* (青金膏 *Blue-Golden Paste*) but the child still had diarrhea for three times, complicated by dry mouth and body fever. Mr. Qi also considered there was mild fever which hadn't subsided completely. Again *Qīngjīngāo* (青金膏 *Blue-Golden Paste*) was prepased and his wife said: "You have applied the medicine for over ten times but the disease is not cured. Can it be that the child has other kinds of disease?" Then Dr. Qian was consulted and he said: "The child's disease has become a deficiency syndrome." As Dr. Qian ordered, big doses of *Báizhúsǎn* (白术散 *Powder of Rhizoma Atractylodis Macrocephalae*) were decocted and the child took the medicine from time to time; later *Xiāngguāyuán* (香瓜圓 *Pill of Fructus Cucumis Sativi*) was applied and the disease was cured after thirteen days.

Case 23

Mr. Cao Xuande's son, at the age of three, had sallow complexion, sometimes chill and fever and only liked to drink water and milk. Many doctors considered it as tidal fever and applied *Niúhuángyuán* (牛黄丸 *Calculus Bovis Pill*) and *Shèxiāngyuán* (麝香圓 *Moschus Pill*) in the treatment in vain. They also prescribed *Zhǐkěsǎn* (止渴乾葛散 *Anti-Thirst Powder of Lobed Kudzuvine Root*) but the child developed vomiting after medication instead. Dr. Qian said: "It should be given *Báibǐngzǐ* (白餅子 *Medicinal White Muffin*) for purgation; and later supplementation of spleen is adopted, and *Xiāojīyuán* (消積圓 *Resolving Food Retention Pill*) is applied to resolve the food retention because it is aggregation of food." Later on the disease was cured as expected. What's the reason for this? The child did not eat but could only drink water, indicating that the food was retained in the tube and could not be digested, leading to stomach cold. It was taking the anti-thirst powder that resulted in reversal Qi of stomach, leading to vomiting; after purging food retention, the disease could be cured.

Part III
Formulas

001

Dàqīnggāo

大青膏

Great Green Paste

Dàqīnggāo (大青膏 *Great Green Paste*) is used to treat wind syndrome caused by heat exuberance in children, which is going to turn to convulsions; if blood and Qi are not full and cannot dominate evil Qi, it will cause convulsions. Though the stool and urine are normal, hot breath from the mouth should be dispersed.

Powder of *Tiānmá* (天麻 *Rhizoma Gastrodiae*) *1 qian* (3 g); powder of raw *Báifùzǐ* (白附子 *Rhizoma Typhonii Gigantei*) *1.5 qian* (4.5 g); *Qīngdài* (青黛 *Indigo Naturalis*) ground into powder, *1 qian* (3 g); *Xiēwěi* (蠍尾 *Cauda Scorpionis*) deprive of toxin, raw and ground into powder, flesh of *Wūshāoshé* (烏梢蛇 *Zaocys*) steeped in wine, baked to dry and ground into powder, *1 qian* (3 g) respectively; *Zhūshā* (硃砂 *Cinnabaris*), *Tiānzhúhuáng* (天竺黃 *Concretio Silicea Bambusae*) ground into powder, and *Shèxiāng* (麝香 *Moschus*) *1 zibi* (0.45 g) respectively.

The ingredients mentioned above are again ground into fine powder and mixed with raw honey into paste; for each

149

dose, a small section of paste as big as *0.5* to *1 zaozi* (皂子 *Semen Gleditsiae Sinensis*), or as a grain of polished japonica rice for the newborn, is taken after being dissolved in warm water of *Niúhuánggāo* (牛黄膏 *Calculus Bovis Paste*) and mint. For the child over five years old, the paste is taken with *Gānlùsǎn* (甘露散 *Sweet Dew Powder*).

002

Liángjīngyuán(wán)

涼驚圓

Fright-Cooling Pill

Liángjīngyuán (涼驚圓 *Fright-Cooling Pill*) is used to treat infantile malnutrition.

Cǎolóngdǎn (草龍膽 *Radix Gentianae*), *Fángfēng* (防風 *Radix Saposhnikoviae*) and *Qīngdài* (青黛 *Indigo Naturalis*) *3 qian* (9 g) respectively; *Gōuténg* (鉤藤 *Ramulus Uncariae Cum Uncis*) *2 qian* (6 g); *Huánglián* (黃連 *Rhizoma Coptidis*) *5 qian* (15 g); *Niúhuáng* (牛黃 *Calculus Bovis*), *Shèxiāng* (麝香 *Moschus*) and *Lóngnǎo* (龍腦 *Borneolum Syntheticum*) *1 zibi* (0.45 g) respectively.

The ingredients mentioned above are ground into powder and mixed with flour to make pill as big as millet; *three–five* to *10–20* pills are taken with water boiled in gold or silver container.

003

Fěnhóngyuán(wán)

粉紅圓

Pink Pill

Fěnhóngyuán (粉紅圓 *Pink Pill*) is also named *Warmly-Relieving-Seizure Pill*.

Zhìtiānnánxīng (炙天南星 *Rhizoma Arisaematis*) is steeped in ox-gall for more than one hundred days during midwinter and dried in the shade, and *4 liang* (120 g) of the powder is taken and ground into fine powder individually. If there is no condition for brewing, raw *Zhìtiānnánxīng* (炙天南星 *Rhizoma Arisaematis*) is filed into powder and stir-fried to ripe for medication.

Zhūshā (硃砂 *Cinnabaris*) *1.5 fen* (4.5 g) ground into powder; *Tiānzhúhuáng* (天竺黃 *Concretio Silicea Bambusae*) *1 liang* (30 g) ground into powder; *Lóngnǎo* (龍腦 *Borneolum Syntheticum*) 0.5 *zi* (0.225 g) ground into powder separately; and *Pēizǐ Yānzhī* (胚子胭脂 *Paste of Primula maximowiczii Regel*) *1 qian* (3 g) ground into powder for applying rouge to the pills.

The ingredients mentioned above are mixed with ox bile to make pill as big as *Qiànshí* (芡實 *Semen Euryales*); for each dose, *1* pill or *0.5* pill for the younger child is taken with granulated sugar dissolved in warm water.

004

Xièqīngyuán(wán)

瀉青圓

Purging-Blue (Liver Heat) Pill

Xièqīngyuán (瀉青圓 *Purging-Blue Pill*) is used to treat any convulsions of hands and feet with surging and excessive pulse due to excessive heat of liver meridian.

Dāngguī (當歸 *Radix Angelicae Sinensis*) deprived of root head and weighed after being sliced, baked to dry; *Lóngdǎn* (龍膽 *Radix Gentianae*) baked to dry and weighed; *Chuānxiōng* (川芎 *Rhizoma Chuanxiong*), *Shānzhī* (山栀子仁 *Fructus Gardeniae*), *Chuāndàhuáng* (川大黃 *Radix et Rhizoma Rhei Palmati*) roasted after being wrapped in wet paper; *Qiānghuó* (羌活 *Rhizoma et Radix Notopterygii*), *Fángfēng* (防風 *Radix Saposhnikoviae*) deprived of root head, sliced and weighed after being baked.

The ingredients mentioned above have the same dosage respectively, and are ground into powder and mixed with refined honey to make pill as big as *Qiànshí* (芡實 *Semen Euryales*); for each dose *0.5* to *1* pill is dissolved in warm sugar water and taken with *Zhúyètāng* (竹葉湯 *Decoction of Olium Phyllostachytis Henonis*).

005

Dìhuángyuán(wán)

地黃圓

Rehmaniae Pill

Dìhuángyuán (地黃圓 *Rehmaniae Pill*) is a formula to treat aphonia, delayed closure of fontanel, lack of spirit, the more whites of both eyes and pale complexion due to insufficiency of kidney Yin.

Shúdìhuáng (熟地黃 *Radix Rehmanniae Preparata*) stir-fried and weighed *8 qian* (24 g); *Shānyúròu* (山萸肉 *Fructus Corni*) and *Gānshānyào* (幹山藥 *Rhizoma Dioscoreae Oppositae*) *4 qian* (12 g) respectively; *Zéxiè* (澤瀉 *Rhizoma Alismatis*), *Mǔdānpí* (牡丹皮 *Cortex Moutan Radicis*) and *Báifúlíng* (白茯苓 *Poria*) deprived of peels, *3 qian* (9 g) respectively.

The ingredients mentioned above are ground into powder and mixed with refined honey to make pill as big as *Wúzǐ* (梧子 *semen firmianae*), and three pills are dissolved in warm water and taken while fasting.

006

Xièbáisăn

瀉白散

Purging White (Lung Heat) Powder

Xièbáisăn (瀉白散 *Purging White Powder*) is also named *Xièfèisăn* (瀉肺散 *Purging lung heat Powder*), and used to treat tachypnea and cough of children due to lung exuberant heat.

Dìgŭpí (地骨皮 *Cortex Lycii Radicis*) deprived of soil and baked to dry, *Sāngbáipí* (桑白皮 *Cortex Mori Albae Radicis*) filed into ends, stir-fried to yellow, *1 liang* (30 g) respectively; *Gāncăo* (甘草 *Radix Glycyrrhizae Preparata*) *1 qian* (3 g).

The ingredients mentioned above are filed into ends and decocted with a pinch of polished japonica rice in two small cups of water till water is left seven in ten and the decoction is taken before meal.

007

Ējiāosǎn

阿膠散

Donkey-Hide Gelatin Powder

Ējiāosǎn (阿膠散 *Donkey-Hide Gelatin Powder*) is also named *Lung-invigorated Powder* (補肺散) and used to treat infantile lung deficiency leading to excessive breathing and panting.

Ējiāo (阿膠 *Colla Corii Asini*) *1 liang and 5 qian* (45 g) stir-fried with bran; *Shǔniánzǐ* (黍粘子 *Semen Panici Miliacei*) stir-fried to fragrance and *Gāncǎo* 甘草 (*Radix Glycyrrhizae Preparata*), 2.5 qian (7.5 g) respectively; *Mǎdōulíng* (馬兜鈴 *Fructus Aristolochiae Debilis*) 5 qian (15 g) baked slightly; seven *Xìngrén* (杏仁 *Semen Armeniacae Amarum*) deprived of skin and spikes and stir-fried; *Nuòmǐ* (糯米 *Oryzae Glutinosae*) *1 liang* (30 g) stir-fried.

The ingredients mentioned above are ground into powder, which is decocted with a cup of water till the water is left six in ten and then taken warmly after meals.

008

Dǎochìsǎn

導赤散

Redness-Purging (Heart Heat) Powder

Dǎochìsǎn (導赤散 *Redness-Purging Powder*) is used to treat infantile excessive heat of heart meridian. The signs by inspection include heat-Qi from the mouth when sleeping, preferring prone position, hyper-strabismus and teeth grinding, which are all due to excessive heat of heart meridian. The heat-Qi of heart meridian leads to the heat of heart and chest and the child wants to speak in vain and prefers the cold so that the child takes the prone position when sleeping.

Shēngdìhuáng (生地黃 *Radix Rehmanniae*), raw *Gāncǎo* (甘草 *Radix Glycyrrhizae*) and *Mùtōng* (木通 *Caulis Akebiae*) with the same dosage respectively.

The ingredients mentioned above are ground into powder and for each dose *3 qian* (9 g) of powder is decocted in a cup of water with *Zhúyè* (竹葉 *Olium Phyllostachytis Henonis*) till the water is left five in ten and taken warmly after meal. In another medical book *Huángqín* (黃芩 *Radix Scutellariae Baicalensis*) is used instead of *Gāncǎo* (甘草 *Radix Glycyrrhizae*).

009

Yìhuángsǎn

益黄散

Benefiting Yellow (Spleen) Powder

Yìhuángsǎn (益黄散 *Benefiting Yellow (Spleen) Powder*) is also termed *Benefiting Spleen Powder* (補脾散) and used to treat spleen deficiency, infantile malnutrition involving spleen, bulging abdomen and thin body.

Chénpí (陳皮 *Pericarpium Citri Reticulatae*) deprived of white pulp, *1 liang* (30 g); *Dīngxiāng* (丁香 *Flos Syzygii Aromatici*) 2 *qian* (6 g), *Mùxiāng* (木香 *Radix Aucklandiae*) is used instead in another formula; *Hēzǐ* (訶子 *Fructus Chebulae*) processed and deprived of nucleus, *Qīngpí* (青皮 *Pericarpium Citri Reticulatae Viride*) deprived of white pulp, *Gāncǎo* 甘草 (*Radix Glycyrrhizae Preparata*), 5 *qian* (15 g) respectively.

The ingredients mentioned above are ground into powder; for the child at the age of over three years old, *1.5 qian* (4.5 g) of the powder is decocted with half a cup of water till the water is left three in ten and taken before meal.

010

Xièhuángsǎn

瀉黃散

Purging-Yellow
(Spleen Heat) Powder

Xièhuángsǎn (瀉黃散 *Purging-Yellow Powder*) has another name *Powder of Purging Spleen Heat* and is used to treat wagging tongue due to spleen heat.

Huòxiāngyè (藿香葉 *Herba Agastaches Rugosae*) *7 qian* (21 g); *Shānzhīrén* (山梔子仁 *Fructus Gardeniae*) *1 qian* (3 g); *Shígāo* (石膏 *Gypsum Fibrosum*) *5 qian* (15 g); *Gāncǎo* (甘草 *Radix Glycyrrhizae*) *3 liang* (90 g); *Fángfēng* (防風 *Radix Saposhnikoviae*) *4 liang* (120 g) deprived of root head, sliced, baked to dry.

The ingredients mentioned above are filed into powder and stir-fried to powder with honey wine; for each dose *1–2 qian* (3–6 g) of the powder is decocted with a cup of water till the water is left five in fen and taken warmly after being filtered anytime.

011

Báizhúsǎn

白術散

Powder of Rhizoma Atractylodis Macrocephalae

Báizhúsǎn （白術散 *Powder of Rhizoma Atractylodis Macrocephalae*) is used to treat frequent vomiting and diarrhea due to long-time deficiency of spleen and stomach, which causes frequent vomiting and diarrhea, exhaustion of essence liquid, vexing thirst for water only, no appetite for breast milk, emaciation and fatigue. With no prompt treatment for a long time, it would turn into fright epilepsy. It is suitable to take the powder whether it is the syndrome of deficiency or excess as well as Yin or Yang.

Rénshēn (人参 *Radix Ginseng*) deprived of root head, *2.5 qian* (7.5 g); *Báifúlíng* （白茯苓 *Poria*) 5 *qian* (15 g); *Báizhú* (白術 *Rhizoma Atractylodis Macrocephalae*) 5 *qian* (15 g), stir-fried; *Huòxiāngyè* (藿香葉 *Herba Agastaches Rugosae*) 5 *qian* (15 g); *Mùxiāng* (木香 *Radix Aucklandiae*) 2 *qian* (6 g); *Gāncǎo* (甘草 *Radix Glycyrrhizae*) 1 *qian* (3 g); and *Gěgēn*

(葛根 *Radix Puerariae Lobatae*) *5 qian* (15 g), double the dosage to *1 liang* (30 g) if feeling thirsty.

The ingredients mentioned above are cut into feeling, and for each dose *3 qian* (9 g) is decocted with water. *Mùxiāng* (木香 *Radix Aucklandiae*) can be taken away if there is dysphoria and thirst due to heat exuberance.

012

Túxìnfǎ

塗囟法

Therapy of Applying Paste Over Fontane

Shèxiāng (麝香 *Moschus*) *1 zibi* (0.45 g); *Xiēwěi* (蠍尾 *Cauda Scorpionis*) deprived of toxin and ground into powder, *0.5 qian* (1.5 g) or *0.5 zibi* (0.225 g) in another formula; *Bóhéyè* (薄荷葉 *Herba Menthae Heplocalycis*) *0.5 zibi* (0.225 g); powder of *Wúgōng* (蜈蚣 *Scolopendra*), *Niúhuáng* (牛黃 *Calculus Bovis*) and *Qīngdài* (青黛 *Indigo Naturalis*) *1 zibi (0.45 g)* respectively.

The ingredients mentioned above are ground together evenly into powder and mixed with the flesh of ripe *Zǎo* (棗 *Fructus Jujubae*) to make a paste, which is smeared over new cotton cloth and stuck on the fontanel; there is a margin by one finger width around the fontanel where the hand presses on fontanel frequently after the hand is warmed over a fire. The therapy is suitable for children at the age of about one hundred days.

013

Yùtǐfǎ

浴體法

Medicinal Bath Therapy

Yùtǐfǎ (浴體法 *Medicinal Bath Therapy*) is used to treat fetal obesity, fetal heat and fetal timidity of children.

Powder of *Tiānmá* (天麻 *Rhizoma Gastrodiae*) *2 qian* (6 g); *Quánxiē* (全蝎 *Scorpio*) deprived of toxin and ground into powder and *Zhūshā* (硃砂 *Cinnabaris*) *5 qian* (15 g) respectively; *Wūshéròu* (烏蛇肉 *Zaocys*) steeped in wine and baked to dry, and *Báifán* (白礬 *Alumen*) *2 qian* (6 g) respectively; *Shèxiāng* (麝香 *Moschus*) *1 qian* (3 g); *Qīngdài* (青黛 *Indigo Naturalis*) *3 qian* (9 g).

The ingredients mentioned above are ground together evenly into powder; for each time *3 qian* (9 g) of powder is decocted in three bowls of water with a bundle of peach branchlets *Táozhī* (桃枝 *Ramulus Persicae*) and five to seven pieces of peach juvenile leaves, and the child has a bath in the warm decoction liquid but his back should be avoided when bathing.

014

Gānjútāng

甘桔湯

Decoction of Liquorice Root and Platycodon Root

Gānjútāng (甘桔湯 *Decoction of Liquorice Root and Platycodon Root*) is used to treat rubbing eyebrows, eyes, nose and face due to lung heat of children.

Jiégěng (桔梗 *Radix Platycodi*) *2 liang* (60 g); *Gāncǎo* (甘草 *Radix Glycyrrhizae*) *1 liang* (30 g).

The ingredients mentioned above are ground into rough powder; for each dose *2 qian* (6 g) of the powder is decocted to seven in ten with a little cup of water and then taken after meal after the decoction is filtered. If *Jīngjiè* (荆芥 *Herba Schizonepetae Tenuifoliae*) and *Fángfēng* (防風 *Radix Saposhnikoviae*) are added to the formula, it is termed *Rúshèngtāng* (*Saint-Like Decoction*). If there is exuberant heat, *Qiānghuó* (羌活 *Rhizoma et Radix Notopterygii*), *Huángqín* (黄芩 *Radix Scutellariae Baicalensis*) and *Shēngmá* (昇麻 *Rhizoma Cimicifugae Foetidae*) are added.

015

Ānshényuán(wán)

安神圓

Mind-Tranquilizing Pill

Ānshényuán (安神圓 *Mind-Tranquilizing Pill*) is used to treat yellowish complexion, red cheek and high body fever due to excessive fire of heart meridian, and can invigorate heart and tranquilize mind. It is also used to treat spiritual trance due to heart deficiency and liver heat.

Mǎyáxiāo (馬牙硝 *Natrii Sulfas*) 5 *qian* (15 g); *Báifúlíng* (白茯苓 *Poria*) 5 *qian* (15 g); *Màiméndōng* (麥門冬 *Radix Ophiopogonis Japonici*) 5 *qian* (15 g); *Gānshānyào* (幹山藥 *Rhizoma Dioscoreae Oppositae*) 5 *qian* (15 g); *Lóngnǎo* (龍腦 *Borneolum Syntheticum*) 1 *zi* (0.45 g) ground into powder; *Hánshuǐshí* (寒水石 *Calcitum*) 5 *qian* (15 g) ground into powder; *Zhūshā* (硃砂 *Cinnabaris*) 1 *liang* (30 g) ground into powder; and *Gāncǎo* (甘草 *Radix Glycyrrhizae*) 5 *qian* (15 g).

The ingredients mentioned above are ground into powder and mixed with refined honey to make pill as big as *Qiànshí* (芡實 *Semen Euryales*); for each dose 0.5 pill dissolved in granulated sugar water is taken anytime.

016

Dāngguīsǎn

當歸散

Powder of Radix Angelicae Sinensis

Dāngguīsǎn (當歸散 *Powder of Radix Angelicae Sinensis*) is used to treat crying at night due to visceral cold causing abdominal pain and also greenish complexion, cold hand and no sucking breast.

Dāngguī (當歸 *Radix Angelicae Sinensis*) deprived of root head, sliced and weighed after being baked to dry, *Báisháoyào* (白芍藥 *Radix Paeoniae Alba*) and *Rénshēn* (人參 *Radix Ginseng*) *1 fen* (0.3 g) respectively; *Gāncǎo* 甘草 (*Radix Glycyrrhizae Preparata*), *0.5 fen* (0.15 g); *Jiégěng* (桔梗 *Radix Platycodi*) and *Chénpí* (陳皮 *Pericarpium Citri Reticulatae*) with the white pulp, *1 fen* (0.3 g) respectively.

The ingredients mentioned above are ground into fine powder and decocted with half a little cup of water, which is taken by a little of dosage anytime. It is taken together with *Sānhuángyuán* (三黃圓 *Three-Yellow Pill*) and *Rénshēntāng* (人參湯 *Ginseng Decoction*) to treat constant crying at midnight, red complexion, dry cracked lips and brown urine.

017

Xièxīntāng

瀉心湯

Purging Heart-Fire Decoction

Xièxīntāng (瀉心湯 *Purging Heart-Fire Decoction*) is used to treat excessive Qi in heart and the difficult movement of Qi up and down; the Qi is not communicated while in prone position so that the child prefers supine position to move Qi up and down smoothly.

Huánglián (黃連 *Rhizoma Coptidis*) *1 liang* (30 g) deprived of branched roots.

The ingredients mentioned above are ground into powder; for each dose *5 fen* (1.5 g) dissolved in warm water is taken before bedtime.

018

Shēngxīsǎn

生犀散

Powder of Raw Rhinoceros Horn

Shēngxīsǎn (生犀散 *Powder of Raw rhinoceros horn*) is used to treat reddish eyes due to deficient heat of heart.

Shēngxījiǎo (生犀角 *Cornu RhinoceriAsiatici*) filed into powder, *2 qian* (6 g); *Dìgǔpí* (地骨皮 *Cortex Lycii Radicis*), better if self-plucked, *Chìsháoyào* (赤芍藥 *Radix Paeoniae Rubra*), *Cháihúgēn* (柴胡根 *Radix Bupleuri Chinensis*) and *Gāngě* (幹葛 *Radix Puerariae Lobatae*) filed into powder, *1 liang* (30 g) respectively; *Gāncǎo* 甘草 (*Radix Glycyrrhizae Preparata*), *5 qian* (15 g).

The ingredients mentioned above are ground into rough powder; for each dose *1–2 qian* (3–6 g) of the powder is decocted with a little cup of water till the water is left seven in ten and taken while the decoction is warm after meal.

019

Báibǐngzǐ

白餅子

Medicinal White Muffin

Báibǐngzǐ (白餅子 *Medicinal White Muffin*) has another name *yùbǐngzǐ* (玉餅子 *Medicinal Jade Muffin*) and is used to treat high fever.

Powders of *Huáshí* (滑石 *Talcum*) *1 qian* (3 g); *Qīngfěn* (輕粉 *Calomelas*) *5 qian* (15 g); powders of *Bànxià* (半夏 *Rhizoma Pinelliae*) *1 qian* (3 g); powders of *Nánxīng* (南星 *Rhizoma Arisaematis*) *1 qian* (3 g); and *24 Bādòu* (巴豆 *Fructus Crotonis*) deprived of skin and membrane; they are boiled in a liter of water till dry and then ground into fine powder.

The first three ingredients are pounded into powder and ground together with *Bādòu* (巴豆 *Fructus Crotonis*) powder first and then with *Qīngfěn* (輕粉 *Calomelas*), which are ground again evenly with remaining powders in the usual way. The final powder is mixed with glutinous rice to make pills as big as mung beans. The dosage is modified according to the deficiency or excess of infant. For the child at the age of less than three years old, *three* to *five* pills are taken while fasting with decoction of *Zǐsū* (紫蘇 *Folium Perillae Zugutae*), avoiding hot food; for the child at the age of three to five years old, the dosage is not given under this limitation and the number of pills can be increased to *20* pills till slight diarrhea develops.

020

Lìjīngyuán(wán)

利驚圓

Fright-Calming Pill

Lìjīngyuán (利驚圓 *Fright-Calming Pill*) is used to treat infantile acute fright wind.

Qīngdài (青黛 *Indigo Naturalis*) and *Qīngfěn* (輕粉 *Calomelas*) *1 qian* (3 g) respectively; powder of *Qiānniú* (牽牛 *Semen Pharbitidis*) *5 qian* (15 g) and *Tiānzhúhuáng* (天竺黃 *Concretio Silicea Bambusae*) *2 qian* (6 g).

The ingredients are ground into powder and mixed with flour to make pills as big as small beans; for each dose *20* pills are taken with mint decoction. In another method, the ingredients are mixed with refined honey to make pills as big as *Qiànshí* (芡實 *Semen Euryales*) and *one* pill is taken after being dissolved.

021

Guālóutāng

栝蔞湯

Decoction of Fructus et Semen Trichosanthis

Guālóutāng (栝蔞湯 *Decoction of Fructus et Semen Trichosanthis*) is used to treat chronic fright.

Guālóugēn (栝蔞根 *Fructus*) *2 qian* (6 g) and *Báigānsuí* (白甘遂 *Radix Kansui*) *1 qian* (3 g).

The ingredients mentioned above are stir-fried over a slow fire to brown and ground evenly; for each dose 1 *zi* (0.45 g) is taken with the decoction of *Shèxiāng* (麝香 *Moschus*) and mint at any time. Any medicine with cold nature will become warm after being stir-fried to brown.

022

Wǔsèyuán(wán)

五色圓

Five Colors Pill

Wǔsèyuán (五色圓 *Five Colors Pill*) is used to treat five kinds of epilepsy.

Zhūshā (硃砂 *Cinnabaris*) *5 qian* (15 g) ground into powder; *Shuǐyín* (水銀 *Hydrargyrum*) *1 liang* (30 g); *Xiónghuáng* (雄黃 *Realgar*) *1 liang* (30 g); and *Qiān* (鉛 *Plumbum*) *3 liang* (90 g) are boiled with *Shuǐyín* (水銀 *Hydrargyrum*); powder of *Zhēnzhū* (珍珠 *Margarita*) *1 liang* (30 g) ground evenly.

The ingredients mentioned above are mixed with refined honey to make pills as big as sesame seeds; for each dose three to four pills are taken with decoction of mint which is decocted in gold or silver container.

023

Tiáozhōngyuán(wán)

調中圓

Middle-Regulating Pill

Tiáozhōngyuán (調中圓 *Middle-Regulating Pill*) is used to treat deficient cold of spleen and stomach, which is also termed *Lǐzhōngyuán* (理中圓 *Regulating Middle-Jiao Yuan*).

Rénshēn (人參 *Radix Ginseng*) deprived of root head, *Báizhú* (白術 *Rhizoma Atractylodis Macrocephalae*) and *Gānjiāng* (乾薑 *Rhizoma Zingiberis*) processed, *3 liang* (90 g) respectively; and *Gāncǎo*甘草 (*Radix Glycyrrhizae Preparata*) *0.5 liang* (15 g).

The ingredients mentioned above are ground into fine powder to make pills as big as mung beans; *0.5* pill to *20–30* pills are taken with warm water before meal.

024

Tāqìyuán(wán)

塌氣圓

Distention-Bleeded Pill

Tāqìyuán (塌氣圓 *Distention-Bleeded Pill*) is used to treat deficient distention. If there is bulging abdomen, *Luóbogēn* (蘿蔔子 *Semen Raphani Sativi*) can be added, which is called *Hèyuánzǐ* (褐圓子 *Brown Pill*).

Hújiāo (胡椒 *Fructus Piperis Nigri*) *1 liang* (30 g) and *Xiēwěi* (蠍尾 *Cauda Scorpionis*) deprived of toxin, *5 qian* (15 g).

The ingredients are ground into fine powder and mixed with flour to make pills as big as millet; for each dose *5–7* to *10–20 pills* are taken with old rice juice anytime. There is *Mùxiāng* (木香 *Radix Aucklandiae*) *1 qian* (3 g) in another formula.

025

Mùxiāngyuán(wán)

木香圓

Costusroot Pill

Mùxiāngyuán (木香圓 *Costusroot Pill*) is used to treat infantile malnutrition with thin body and bulging abdomen.

Mùxiāng (木香 *Radix Aucklandiae*) and *Qīngdài* (青黛 *Indigo Naturalis*) ground individually, *Bīngláng* (檳榔 *Semen Arecae*) and *Dòukòu* (豆蔻 *Fructus Amomi Rotundus*) peeled, *1 fen* (0.3 g) respectively; *Shèxiāng* (麝香 *Moschus*) ground individually, *1.5 fen* (0.45 g); *Xùsuízi* (續隨子 *Semen Euphorbia*) peeled, *1 liang* (30 g); three *Xiāmá* (蝦蟆 *Rana Siccus*) burnt with preserving nature.

The ingredients are ground into fine powder and mixed with honey to make pills as big as mung beans; for each dose *3–5* to *10–20 pills* are taken with mint decoction before meal.

026

Húhuángliányuán(wán)

胡黄連圓

Pill of Rhizoma Picrorhizae

Húhuángliányuán (胡黄連圓 *Pill of Rhizoma Picrorhizae*) is used to treat infantile malnutrition involving spleen with fatness and fever.

Chuānhuánglián (川黄連 *Rhizoma Coptidis*) *5 qian* (15 g); *Húhuánglián* (胡黄連 *Rhizoma Picrorhizae*) *5 qian* (15 g); *Zhūshā* (硃砂 *Cinnabaris*) *1 qian* (3 g), ground individually.

The first two ingredients are ground into fine powder and together with powder of *Zhūshā* (硃砂 *Cinnabaris*), which are put into *Zhūdǎn* (豬膽 *Fellis Suillus or pig gallbladder*) and boiled in malting liquid; the gallbladder is hung by a thread from a wood stick over a medicinal pot but doesn't touch the bottom of the pot; after waiting for about a meal's time, the gallbladder is taken out, ground together with *Lúhuì* (蘆薈 *Aloe*) and *Shèxiāng* (麝香 *Moschus*) *1 fen* (0.3 g) respectively and mixed with cooked rice to make pills as big as sesame seeds; for each dose *5–7 to 20–30 pills* are taken with rice liquid after meal.

027

Lánxiāngsǎn

蘭香散

Powder of Herba seu Radix Caryopteridis Incanae

Lánxiāngsǎn (蘭香散 *Powder of Herba seu Radix Caryopteridis Incanae*) is used to treat evil Qi due to infantile malnutrition and red ulceration of lower part of the nose.

Lánxiāng (蘭香 *Herba seu Radix Caryopteridis Incanaem; vegetable*) burnt with preserving nature, *2 qian* (6 g); *Tóngqīng* (銅青 *Mineralium Viridianum*) *5 fen* (1.5 g) and *Qīngfěn* (輕粉 *Calomelas*) *2 zi* (0.9 g).

The ingredients are ground into fine powder and stirred evenly, and according to the area of the spot, the proper dosage of the powder is applied on it.

028

Báifěnsǎn

白粉散

The Whites Powder

Báifěnsǎn (白粉散 *The Whites Powder*) is used to treat the sore due to infantile malnutrition.

Hǎipiāoshāo (海螵蛸 *Os Sepiellae seu Sepiae*) *3 fen* (0.9 g); *Báijí* (白及 *Rhizoma Bletillae Striatae*) *3 fen* (0.9 g) and *Qīngfěn* (輕粉 *Calomelas*) *1 fen* (0.3 g).

The ingredients are ground into fine powder; the sore is first washed with malting liquid and then the powder is applied after the sore is dry.

029

Xiāojīyuán(wán)

消積圓

Resolving Food Retention Pill

Xiāojīyuán (消積圓 *Resolving Food Retention Pill*) is used to treat stool with sour smell due to food retention.

Nine pieces of *Dīngxiāng* (丁香 *Flos Syzygii Aromatici*); *20 pieces* of *hārén* (縮砂仁 *FructusAmomi Villosi*) and *3 pieces of Wūméiròu* (烏梅肉 *Fructus Mume*) baked to dry; *2 Bādòu* (巴豆 *Fructus Crotonis*) baked and deprived of skin, oil, core and membrane.

The ingredients mentioned above are ground into fine powder and mixed with flour to make pills as big as millet. For children at the age of over three years old, *3–5* pills; *2–3* pills for younger than three years old, taken with warm water at any time.

030

Ānchóngsǎn

安蟲散

Parasite-Expelling Powder

Ānchóngsǎn (安蟲散 *Parasite-Expelling Powder*) is used to treat abdominal pain due to worm disease.

Húfěn (胡粉 *Hydrocerussitum*) stir-fried to yellow, *Bīngláng* (檳榔 *Semen Arecae*) and *Chuānliànzǐ* (川楝子 *Fructus Toosendan*) deprived of skin and nucleus, *Hèshī* (鶴虱 *Fructus Carpesii*) burnt to yellow, *2 liang* (60 g) respectively, and *Báifán* (白礬 *Alumen*) boiled in iron pot, *1 fen* (0.3 g).

The ingredients are ground into fine powder; for each dose *1 zi* (0.45 g) or *0.5 qian* (1.5 g) for elder child, is taken with warm rice juice when the abdominal pain attacks.

031

Zǐshuāngyuán(wán)

紫霜圓

Purple Cream Pill

Zǐshuāngyuán (紫霜圓 *Purple Cream Pill*) is used to dissipate local accumulation and aggregation.

Dàizhěshí (代赭石 *Haematitum*) calcined and quenched in vinegar for seven times, and *Chìshízhī* (赤石脂 *Halloysitum Rubrum*), *1 qian* (3 g) respectively; *50 Xìngrén* (杏仁 *Semen Armeniacae Amarum*) deprived of skin and spikes; *30 Bādòu* (巴豆 *Fructus Crotonis*) deprived of skin, core and oil.

First *Xìngrén* (杏仁 *Semen Armeniacae Amarum*) and *Bādòushuāng* (巴豆霜 *Semen Crotonis Pulveratum*) are put into a porcelain mortar and ground finely till paste is formed; additionally powder of *Dàizhěshí* (代赭石 *Haematitum*) and *Chìshízhī* (赤石脂 *Halloysitum Rubrum*) are put into the porcelain mortar and ground evenly, which is then mixed with steamed cake steeped in hot water to make pills as big as millet. For children at the age of one year old, *five* pills are taken with rice juice; for children at the age of 100–200 days, *three* pills are taken with milk. The dosage is modified according to the condition of excess or deficiency till slight diarrhea develops. The pills are also used to treat many diseases concerned with fright due to phlegm, and though it is a purging therapy, it has no risk of causing deficiency.

032

Zhǐhànsǎn

止汗散

Anti-Perspiration Powder

Zhǐhànsǎn (止汗散 *Anti-Perspiration Powder*) is used to treat deficient sweating due to infantile exuberant heat, from the head to nape but not through the chest and it needn't be treated. The child tends to sweat frequently and has profuse sweating on the frontal head while wearing thick clothes during sleep, and it is treated mainly with *Zhǐhànsǎn* (止汗散 *Anti-Perspiration Powder*).

An old and broken fan made of cattail leaf is out of shape and is burnt to ashes: *Púshànhuī* (蒲扇灰 ashes of *Cattail Leaf Fan*).

The ashes mentioned above are ground finely and for each dose *1–2 qian* (3–6 g) is taken with warm wine at any time.

033

Xiāngguāyuán(wán)

香瓜圓

Fragrant Cucumber Pill

Xiāngguāyuán (香瓜圓 *Fragrant Cucumber Pill*) is used to treat sweating all over the body due to excess heat of heart.

One big *Huánggguā* (黃瓜 *Fructus Cucumis Sativi*) with yellow color, deprived of pulp; *Chuāndàhuáng* (川大黃 *Radix et Rhizoma Rhei Palmati*) wrapped in wet paper and roasted till the paper is charred; *Húhuánglián* (胡黃連 *Rhizoma Picrorhizae*), *Cháihú* (柴胡 *Radix Bupleuri Chinensis*) deprived of root head, *Biējiǎ* (鱉甲 *Carapax Trionycis*) with vinegar burnt over a slow fire till it becomes yellow, *Lúhuì* (蘆薈 *Aloe*), *Qīngpí* (青皮 *Pericarpium Citri Reticulatae Viride*), *Huángbò* (黃檗 *Phellodendron amurense Rupr.*) and *Huánglián* (黃連 *Rhizoma Coptidis*) with the same dosage respectively.

Except for *Huánggguā* (黃瓜 *Fructus Cucumis Sativi*), the ingredients mentioned above are ground together into fine powder; the head of *Huánggguā* (黃瓜 *Fructus Cucumis Sativi*) is removed, the fine powder is put into the *Huánggguā* (黃瓜 *Fructus Cucumis Sativi*) fully, the hole is covered with the head and is fixed with pegwood; it is roasted over a slow fire till soft and then mixed with flour to make pills as big as mung beans. For each dose *two* to *three* pills are taken with cold malting water or fresh well water; for elder children, *five, seven* to *10* pills can be taken.

034

Huāhuǒgāo

花火膏

Candlewick Powder

Huāhuǒgāo (花火膏 *Candlewick Powder*) is used to treat night crying.

One piece of burnt *Dēnghuā* (燈花 *Candlewick*).

The wick is taken down from the oil lamp and its ash is smeared on the nipple, and then let the baby suck the milk.

035

Báiyùsǎn

白玉散

White-Jade-Like Powder

Báiyùsǎn (白玉散 *White-Jade-Like Powder*) is used to treat toxic invasion of toxic heat into interstitial striae and struggling of blood and Qi to erupt in the skin with red color like cinnabar; it is used as an ushering formula.

Báitǔ (白土 *Calcium Carbonate*) 2.5 *qian* (7.5 g) with another name *Huáshí* (滑石 *Talcum*), and *Hánshuǐshí* (寒水石 *Calcitum*) 5 *qian* (15 g).

The ingredients mentioned above are ground into fine powder and mixed with vinegar or fresh well water, and then applied on the spot.

036

Niúhuánggāo

牛黄膏

Calculus Bovis Paste

Niúhuánggāo (牛黃膏 *Calculus Bovis Paste*) is used to treat febrile fright.

Xiónghuáng (雄黃 *Realgar*) as big as a small Jujube is boiled in a mug of water containing the juice of *Luóbogēn* (蘿蔔根 *Semen Raphani Sativi*) and *Cù* (醋 *Vinegar*); powder of *Gāncǎo* (甘草 *Radix Glycyrrhizae*) and *Tiánxiāo* (甜硝 *Sweet Mirabilite*), *3 qian* (9 g) respectively; *Zhūshā* (硃砂 *Cinnabaris*) 0.5 qianbi (0.9 g) and *Lóngnǎo* (龍腦 *Borneolum Syntheticum*) *1 qianbi* (1.8 g); *Hánshuǐshí* (寒水石 *Calcitum*) ground into fine powder, *5 qianbi* (9 g).

The ingredients are ground evenly and mixed with honey to make pills; the paste as big as *0.5 zaozi* (皂子 *Semen Gleditsiae Sinensis*) is dissolved in warm mint decoction and taken after meal.

037

Niúhuángyuán(wán)

牛黃圓

Pill of Calculus Bovis

Niúhuángyuán (牛黃圓 *Pill of Calculus Bovis*) is used to treat food retention due to infantile malnutrition.

Xiónghuáng (雄黃 *Realgar*) ground with water, and *Tiānzhúhuáng* (天竺黃 *Concretio SiliceaBambusae*) *2 qian* (6 g) respectively; powder of *Qiānniú* (牽牛 *Semen Pharbitidis*) *1 qian* (3 g).

The ingredients mentioned above are again ground together and mixed with flour to make pills as big as millet; for each dose *three* to *five* pills are taken after meal with mint decoction. It is also used to treat infantile malnutrition and to dissipate food retention, and has better effect if taken frequently and the number of pills is increased for elder children.

038

Yùlùsǎn

玉露散

Jade-Dew Powder

Yùlùsǎn (玉露散 *Jade-Dew Powder*) has another name *Gānlùsǎn* (甘露散 *Sweet Dew Powder*) and is used to treat vomiting, diarrhea, sallow and thin body due to heat evil damaging viscera.

Hánshuǐshí (寒水石 *Calcitum*) is soft with slight blue-black color and with fine texture; *Shígāo* (石膏 *Gypsum Fibrosum*) is hard and white with flat shape and has good quality if it cannot be broken; 0.5 *liang* (15 g) respectively; and raw *Gāncǎo* (甘草 *Radix Glycyrrhizae*) 1 *qian* (3 g).

The ingredients are made into fine powder; for each dose 1 *zi* (0.45 g), 0.5 *qian* (1.5 g) or 1 *qian* (3 g) is taken with warm water after meal.

039

Bǎixiángyuán(wán)

百祥圓

Hundred-Luck Pill

Bǎixiángyuán (百祥圓 *Hundred-Luck Pill*) has another name called *Nanyangyuán* (南陽圓 *Nanyang Pill*) and is used to treat sore and rash, ulcerative spot or black depression.

The definite dosage of *Hóngyádàjǐ* (红芽大戟 *Radix Knoxiae*) is dried in the shade and boiled with malt liquid to remove hard parts when it is soft; later it is dried under the burning sun; then it is boiled again with the liquid till no juice is left and baked dry; its powder is mixed with water to make pills as big as millet; for each dose *10* to *20* pills are taken with decoction of ground sesames till vomiting and diarrhea have stopped and it can be taken anytime.

040

Niúlǐgāo

牛李膏

Paste of Radix Seu Cortex Rhamnus utilis

Niúlǐgāo (牛李膏 *Paste of Radix Seu Cortex Rhamnus utilis*) is a byname for *Bìshènggāo* (必胜膏 *Succeeding Paste*), and its usage is the same as the previous *Bǎixiángyuán* (百祥圓 *Hundred-Luck Pill*).

041

Niúlǐzǐ

牛李子

Fructus Rhamnus Davuricae

The fruits are pounded in a stone mortar and the powder is boiled into paste; for each dose the paste as much as *1 zaozi* (皂子 *Semen Gleditsiae Sinensis*) is dissolved in *Xìngjiāotāng* (杏膠湯 *Decoction of Semen Armeniacae Amarum and Colla Corii Bovis*) and taken.

042

Xuānfēngsǎn

宣風散

Wind-Dispersing Powder

Xuānfēngsǎn (宣風散 *Wind-Dispersing Powder*) is used to treat infantile chronic fright.

Two *Bīngláng* (槟榔 *Semen Arecae*), *Chénpí* (陳皮 *Pericarpium Citri Reticulatae*) and *Gāncǎo* (甘草 *Radix Glycyrrhizae*) 0.5 liang (15 g) respectively; half-ripe and half-raw *Qiānniúzǐ* (牽牛 *Semen Pharbitidis*) 4 liang (120 g).

The ingredients mentioned above are ground into fine powder. For children at the age of 2–3 years old, *5 fen* (1.5 g) of powder dissolved in honey soup is taken, or *1 qian* (3 g) for children at the age of over 2–3 years old is taken before meal.

043

Shèxiāngyuán(wán)

麝香圓

Moschus Pill

Shèxiāngyuán (麝香圓 *Moschus Pill*) is used to treat any fright and infantile malnutrition.

Cǎolóngdǎn (草龍膽 *Radix Gentianae*) and *Húhuánglián* (胡黃連 *Rhizoma Picrorhizae*) 0.5 *liang* (15 g) respectively; *Mùxiāng* (木香 *Radix Aucklandiae*) and *Chántuì* (蟬殼 *Periostracum Cryptotympanae*) deprived of spines, made into powder and weighed after being dried, *Lúhuì* (蘆薈 *Aloe*) deprived of sand and weighed, *Xióngdǎn* (熊膽 *Fel Selenarcti*) and *Qīngdài* (青黛 *Indigo Naturalis*) 1 *qian* (3 g) respectively; *Qīngfěn* (輕粉 *Calomelas*), *Nǎoshè* (脑麝 *Borneolum Syntheticum & Moschu*) and *Niúhuáng* (牛黃 *Calculus Bovis*) 1 *qian* (3 g) respectively, ground into powder individually; 21 pieces of *Guādì* (瓜蒂 *Pedicellus Melo*) made into fine powder.

The ingredients mentioned above are mixed with pig bile to make pills as big as seeds of tung tree or as mung beans; for convulsions associated with infantile malnutrition, constipation or diarrhea due to visceral disoders, 5–7 to 10–20 pills are taken with rice juice or warm water; for infantile malnutrition involving eyes (equivalent to keratomalacia), the pills are taken with pig liver soup; for thirst due to infantile malnutrition, the pills are taken with pork soup or soup of pork with skin; for fright wind, convulsions and hypertropia, *1* pill dissolved in mint decoction is taken and additionally *1* pill is ground in water to drop into the nose; for gingival malnutrition and mouth sore, the pills are ground into powder to apply on the affected part; for abdominal pain due to worm disease, the pills are taken with the decoction of *Kǔliàngēn* (苦楝根 *Cortex Meliae Azedarach*) or *Báiwúyí* (白蕪荑 *Pasta Ulmi*). For infants at the age of less than 100 days with excretive retention, the pills are ground with water to apply on the nave; for manifestation of worm disease, a few *Gānqī* (幹漆 *Resina Toxicodendri*) and good *Shèxiāng* (麝香 *Moschus*) together with 1–2 drops of raw oil are added to the pills, and the medicine is taken after being dissolved in warm water. The pills should be smashed for any acute diseases and should be dissolved for chronic diseases. It is not allowed for infants with extreme deficiency or chronic fright and it is especially suitable for acute fright and phlegm heat.

044

Dàxīngxīngyuán(wán)

大惺惺圓

Big Alerting Pill

Dàxīngxīngyuán (大惺惺圓 *Big Alerting Pill*) is used to treat fright, infantile malnutrition and various diseases as well as diseases due to improper treatment, which are difficult to introduce in detail here.

Chénshā (辰砂 *Cinnabaris*) ground into powder, *Qīngméngshí* (青礞石 *Lapis Chloriti*) and *Jīnyáshí* (金牙石 *Vermiculitum*) *1.5 qian* (4.5 g) respectively; *Xiónghuáng* (雄黃 *Realgar*) *1 qian* (3 g), *Chánhuī* (蟾灰 *Succys Bufo*) *2 qian* (6 g), *Niúhuáng* (牛黃 *Calculus Bovis*) and *Lóngnǎo* (龍腦 *Borneolum Syntheticum*) respectively *1 zi* (0.45 g), ground individually; *Shèxiāng* (麝香 *Moschus*) *0.5 qian (1.5 g)*, ground individually; and *Shéhuáng* (蛇黃 *Radix Paeoniae Alba*) *3 qian* (9 g) quenched in vinegar for five times.

The ingredients mentioned above are ground evenly into fine powder and later boiled in water, which is mixed with steamed cake to make pills with *Zhūshā* (硃砂 *Cinnabaris*) as coating, as big as Mung beans. One pill for infants at the age of less than 100 days and two pills for infants at the age of one year old are taken after meal by dissolving the pills in warm mint decoction.

045

Xiǎoxīngxīngyuán(wán)

小惺惺圓

Small Alerting Pill

Xiǎoxīngxīngyuán (小惺惺圓 *Small Alerting Pill*) is used to detoxify toxin and treat acute fright, wind epilepsy and tidal fever as well as deficient vexation, medicinal toxin attacking upwards and vexing thirst.

The feces of a female pig walking towards the east are collected in winter months and burnt to ash with the nature preserved, *Chénshā* (辰砂 *Cinnabaris*) ground with water, *Nǎoshè* (腦麝 *Borneolum Syntheticum & Moschu*) *2 qian* (6 g) respectively; *Niúhuáng* (牛黃 *Calculus Bovis*) *1 qian* (3 g), ground into powder individually; *Shéhuáng* (蛇黃 *Pyritum Globuloforme*) from Xishan burnt to red, quenched in vinegar for three times, ground with water and dried, *0.5 liang* (15 g).

The ingredients mentioned above are mixed with flour and water flowing east to make pills as big as seeds of tung tree with *Zhūshā* (硃砂 *Cinnabaris*) as coating; for each dose *two* pills for the child at the age of 2–3 years old are taken with warm water after meal when the pills are broken by keys. For the newborn just after birth, it is better to take *one* pill to get rid of many diseases.

046

Yínshāyuán(wán)

銀砂圓

Pill of Hydrargyrum and Cinnabaris

Yínshāyuán (銀砂圓 *Pill of Hydrargyrum and Cinnabaris*) is used to treat profuse spittle, heat in the diaphragm, cough with excessive phlegm, wind fright, food retention and tidal fever.

Shuǐyín (水银 *Hydrargyrum*) formed into particles as big as *three zaozi* (皂子 *Semen Gleditsiae Sinensis*); ground *Chénshā* (辰砂 *Cinnabaris*), 2 *qian* (6 g); *Xiēwěi* (蠍尾 *Cauda Scorpionis*) deprived of toxin and ground into powder; *Péngshā* (硼砂 *Borax*) and *Fěnshuāng* (粉霜 *Mercury Bichloride*) ground respectively; *Qīngfěn* (輕粉 *Calomelas*) and *Yùlǐrén* (郁李仁 *Semen Pruni Japonicae*) peeled and weighed after being baked, which is made into powder; *Báiqiānniú* (白牽牛 *Semen Pharbitidis*), *Tiěfěn* (鐵粉 *Iron Powder*) and good tea collected in the winter (好腊茶), 3 *qian* (9 g) respectively.

The ingredients mentioned above are made into fine powder and boiled with pear juice to make pills as big as green beans. *One* to *three* pills are dissolved with *Bīngpiàn* (冰片 *Borneolum Syntheticum*) in water. The pills have another name called *Lízhī Bǐngzǐ* (梨汁餅子 *Cake of Pear Juice*) and are taken after meal to treat wind spittle in adults.

047

Shéhuángyuán(wán)

蛇黃圓

Pill of Pyritum Globuloforme

Shéhuángyuán (蛇黃圓 *Pill of Pyritum Globuloforme*) is used to treat epilepsy, including manifestations like crying or trance, which is caused by shock or fright.

Three pieces of real *Shéhuáng* (蛇黃 *Pyritum Globuloforme*) calcined and quenched in vinegar; *Yùjīn* (郁金 *Radix Curcumae Wenyujin*) *7 fen* (2.1 g) made into powder together; *Shèxiāng* (麝香 *Moschus*) *1 zibi* (0.45 g).

The ingredients mentioned above are made into powder and mixed with cooked rice to make pills as big as seeds of tung tree. For each dose *1* or *2* pills are taken after being dissolved in water cooked in golden or silver container or sharpening water.

048

Sānshèngyuán(wán)

三聖圓

Three-Saint Pill

Sānshèngyuán (三聖圓 *Three-Saint Pill*) is used to resolve phlegm and spittle, relax the chest and diaphragm and disperse breast lump as well as to relieve fright wind, epilepsy due to too much food and various infantile malnutrition. For infants less than one year old, frequent medication has wonderful effect.

Xiǎoqīngyuán (小青圓 *Little Blue Pill*):
Qīngdài (青黛 *Indigo Naturalis*) *1 qian* (3 g), the powder of *Qiānniúzǐ* (牽牛 *Semen Pharbitidis*), *3 qian* (9 g) and *Nìfěn* (膩粉 *Calomelas*) *1 qian* (3 g).
They are ground together and mixed with flour to make pills as big as millet.

Xiǎohóng yuán (小紅圓 *Little Red Pill*):
Powder of raw *Tiānnánxīng* (天南星 *Rhizoma Arisaematis*), *1 liang* (30 g); *Zhūshā* (硃砂 *Cinnabaris*) *0.5 liang* (15 g),

ground with *Bādòu* (巴豆 *Fructus Crotonis*) *1 qian* (3 g) to take its cream.

They are ground together and mixed with ginger juice and flour to make pills as big as millet.

Xiǎohuáng yuán (小黃圓 *Little Yellow Pill*):

Powder of raw *Bànxià* (半夏 *Rhizoma Pinelliae*) *1 fen* (0.3 g), *Bādòushuāng* (巴豆霜 *Semen Crotonis Pulveratum*), *1 zibi* (0.45 g) and powder of *Huángbò* (黃檗 *Phellodendron amurense Rupr*) *1 zibi* (0.45 g),

They are ground together with ginger juice and flour to make pills as big as millet.

One pill is taken for infants at the age of 100 days and *2* pills are taken with milk for infants at the age of one year old.

049

Tiěfěnyuán(wán)

鐵粉圓

Iron-Powder Pill

Tiěfěnyuán (鐵粉圓 *Iron-powder Pill*) is used to treat profuse drooling, tidal fever, convulsions and vomiting due to reversal Qi.

Shuǐyín (水銀 *Hydrargyrum*) particles, *3 fen* (0.9 g); *Zhūshā* (硃砂 *Cinnabaris*) and *Tiěfěn* (鐵粉 *Ferrous Pulveres*), *1 fen* (0.3 g) respectively; *Qīngfěn* (輕粉 *Calomelas*), *2 fen* (0.6 g); *Tiānnánxīng* (天南星 *Rhizoma Arisaematis*) processed and deprived of rinds and pedicel and ground into powder, *1 fen* (0.3 g).

The ingredients mentioned above are ground together to the extent of not seeing the mercury droplets. Then they are mixed with ginger juice and flour to make pills as big as millet. *Ten* to *15* pills or *20* to *30* pills are taken with decoction of ginger anytime.

050

Yínyèyuán(wán)

銀液圓

Hydrargyrum Pill

Yínyèyuán (銀液圓 *Hydrargyrum Pill*) is used to treat febrile fright and vomiting due to excessive evil in the diaphragm, vomiting and heat drooling and exuberant heat surging upward.

Shuǐyín (水銀 *Hydrargyrum*), *0.5 liang* (15 g); *Tiānnánxīng* (天南星 *Rhizoma Arisaematis*) processed, *2 qian* (6 g); *Báifùzǐ* (白附子 *Rhizoma Typhonii Gigantei*) processed, *1 qian* (3 g).

The ingredients mentioned above are ground into powder, which is mixed with *shínǎoyóu* (石腦油 *Grude oil*) to make pills. For each dose the paste as big as one *zaozi* (皂子 seed of *Chinese Honeylocust*) is taken with decoction of mint.

051

Zhènxīnyuán(wán)

鎮心圓

Heart-Tranquilizing Pill

Zhènxīnyuán (鎮心圓 *Heart-Tranquilizing Pill*) is used to treat epileptic fright and heart heat.

Zhūshā (硃砂 *Cinnabaris*), *Lóngchǐ* (龍齒 *Dens Draconis*) and *Niúhuáng* (牛黃 *Calculus Bovis*) *1 qian* (3 g) respectively; *Tiěfěn* (鐵粉 *Ferrous Pulveres*), *Hǔpò* (琥珀 *Succinum*), *Rénshēn* (人參 *Radix Ginseng*), *Fúlíng* (茯苓 *Poria*) and *Fángfēng* (防風 *Radix Saposhnikoviae*), *2 qian* (6 g) respectively; *7 Quánxiē* (全蝎 *Scorpio*) baked.

The ingredients are ground into powder and mixed with refined honey to make pills as big as seeds of tung tree; for each dose *1* pill is taken with decoction of mint.

052

Jīnbóyuán(wán)

金箔圓

Gold Leaf Pill

Jīnbóyuán(wán) (金箔圓 *Gold Leaf Pill*) is used to treat acute fright with profuse drool.

Twenty pieces of *Jīnbó* (金箔 *Gold Foil*), *Tiānnánxīng* (天南星 *Rhizoma Arisaematis*) filed and stir-fried, *Báifùzǐ* (白附子 *Rhizoma Typhonii Gigantei*) processed, *Fángfēng* (防風 *Radix Saposhnikoviae*) baked after being deprived of head and branched root, *Bànxià* (半夏 *Rhizoma Pinelliae*) steeped in boiling water for seven times, sliced and weighed after baking to dry, *0.5 liang* (15 g) respectively; *Xiónghuáng* (雄黃 *Realgar*) and *Chénshā* (辰砂 *Cinnabaris*), *1 fen* (0.3 g) respectively; powder of *Shēngxī* (生犀 *Cornu Rhinoceri Asiatici*) *0.5 fen* (0.15 g); *Niúhuáng* (牛黃 *Calculus Bovis*) and *Nǎoshè* (龍腦 *Borneolum Syntheticum* & 麝香 *Moschus*) *0.5 fen* (0.15 g) respectively; these ingredients are ground into powder.

The ingredients are ground into fine powder and mixed with ginger juice and flour to make pills as big as sesame seeds; *3–5* to *10–20* pills are taken with ginseng decoction. For chronic fright, *Nǎoshè* (龍腦 *Borneolum Syntheticum*) is removed; the pills are taken anytime.

053

Chénshāyuán(wán)

辰砂圓

Cinnabaris Pill

Chénshāyuán (辰砂圓 *Cinnabaris Pill*) is used to treat fright wind with profuse drool and periodic convulsions as well as constant vomiting and diarrhea due to stomach heat.

Chénshā (辰砂 *Cinnabaris*) ground individually, *Shuǐyín* (水銀 *Hydrargyrum*) granules, *1 fen* (0.3 g) respectively; *Tiānmá* (天麻 *Rhizoma Gastrodiae*) and *Niúhuáng* (牛黃 *Calculus Bovis*) *5 fen* (1.5 g) respectively; *Nǎoshè* (龍腦 *Borneolum Syntheticum* & *Shèxiāng* 麝香 *Moschus*), ground individually, *5 fen* (1.5 g); powder of *Shēngxījiǎo* (生犀 *Cornu Rhinoceri Asiatici*), *Báijiāngcán* (白僵蠶 *Bombyx Batryticatus*) stir-fried in wine, *Chánké* (蟬殼 *Periostracum Cryptotympanae*) deprived of feet, *Gānxiē* (幹蠍 *Scorpionis*) deprived of toxin and stir-fried, *Máhuáng* (麻黃 *Herbaephedrae Sinicae*) deprived of joint and *Tiānnánxīng* (天南星 *Rhizoma Arisaematis*) steeped in boiling water for seven times, sliced and weighed after being baked to dry, *1 fen* (0.3 g) respectively.

The ingredients are ground together and ground again evenly into powder and mixed with ripe honey to make pills as big as mung beans with *Zhūshā* (硃砂 *Cinnabaris*) as coating of pills; *1–2* to *5–7* pills are taken with mint decoction after meal.

054

Jiǎndāogǔyuán(wán)

剪刀股圓

Pill of Herba Ixeritis Japonicae

Jiǎndāogǔyuán (剪刀股圓 *Pill of Herba Ixeritis Japonicae*) is used to treat any fright wind, especially the fright due to deficiency after long-term medication of dispersing and soothing agents.

Zhūshā (硃砂 *Cinnabaris*) and *Tiānzhúhuáng* (天竺黃 *Concretio Silicea Bambusae*) ground into powder individually, *Báijiāngcán* (白僵蠶 *Bombyx Batryticatus*) deprived of head and feet and stir-fried, *Xiē* (蠍 *Scorpio*) deprived of toxin and stir-fried, *Gānchán* (幹蟾 *Succys Bufo*) deprived of four limbs and intestines, washed and stir-fried with adjuvant to brown into powder, *Chánké* (蟬殼 *Periostracum Cicadae*) deprived of spikes and *Wǔlíngzhī* (五靈脂 *Faeces Trogopterori*) deprived of the yellow part and ground into powder, *1 fen* (0.3 g) respectively; *Niúhuáng* (牛黃 *Calculus Bovis*) and *Lóngnǎo* (龍腦 *Borneolum Syntheticum*) ground together into powder, *1 zi* (0.45 g) respectively; *Shèxiāng* (麝香 *Moschus*) ground *5 fen* (1.5 g); *Shéhuáng* (蛇黃 *Pyritum Globuloforme*) *5 qian* (15 g) burnt to red, quenched in vinegar for 3–5 times and ground with water.

The ingredients mentioned above are made into powder, with total amount of *2 liang* and *4 qian* (72 g); the powder is boiled in water from river flowing east and then mixed with white flour to make pills as big as seeds of tung tree; for each dose *1* pill is broken with scissors and taken with mint decoction after meal. For chronic fright *Lóngnǎo* (龍腦 *Borneolum Syntheticum*) is removed.

055

Shèchányuán(wán)

麝蟾圓

Pill of Moschus and Succys Bufo

Shèchányuán (麝蟾圓 *Pill of Moschus and Succys Bufo*) is used to treat fright wind, heat drooling and periodic convulsions.

Big *Gānchán* (幹蟾 *Succys Bufo*) weighed, *2 qian* (6 g), burnt to ash and ground individually; *Tiěfěn* (鐵粉 *Ferrous Pulveres*) *3 qian* (9 g); *Zhūshā* (硃砂 *Cinnabaris*), powder of *Qīngméngshí* (青礞石 *Lapis Chloriti*), powder of *Xiónghuáng* (雄黃 *Realgar*) and *Shéhuáng* (蛇黃 *Pyritum Globuloforme*) burnt and quenched into powder, *2 qianbi* (3.6 g) respectively, *Lóngnǎo* (龍腦 *Borneolum Syntheticum*) *1 zi* (0.45 g); *Shèxiāng* (麝香 *Moschus*) *1 qianbi* (1.8 g).

The ingredients mentioned above are ground evenly, immersed in water and mixed with steamed cake to make pills as big as seeds of tung tree with *Zhūshā* (硃砂 *Cinnabaris*) as pill coating; *0.5* pill or *1* pill is taken with mint decoction at any time.

056

Ruǎnjīndān

軟金丹

Metal-Softening Elixir

Ruǎnjīndān (軟金丹 *Metal-Softening Elixir*) is used to treat febrile fright with profuse phlegm, productive cough and excessive Qi in diaphragm.

Tiānzhúhuáng (天竺黃 *Concretio Silicea Bambusae*) and *Qīngfěn* (輕粉 *Calomelas*) *2 liang* (60 g) respectively; *Qīngdài* (青黛 *Indigo Naturalis*) *1 qian* (3 g); *Hēiqiānniú* (黑牽牛 *Semen Pharbitidis*) ground into powder which is firstly formed, *Bànxià* (半夏 *Rhizoma Pinelliae*) with *Shēngjiāng* (生薑 *Rhizoma Zingiberis Recens*) *3 qian* (9 g) is pounded with leaven, baked to dry and ground again into fine powder, *3 fen* (0.9 g) respectively.

The ingredients mentioned above are ground evenly together and mixed with refined honey to make paste; *0.5 to 1 zaozi* (皂子 *Semen Gleditsiae Sinensis*) of the paste dissolved in mint decoction is taken after meal; the dosage is modified with the age of the child.

057

Táozhīyuán(wán)

桃枝圓

Pill of Ramulus Persicae

Táozhīyuán (桃枝圓 *Pill of Ramulus Persicae*) is used to disperse accumulative heat and chest congestion and it is also known by the name *Táofúyuán* (桃符圓 *Pill of Peach Wood Charm*).

Bādòushuāng (巴豆霜 *Semen Crotonis Pulveratum*), *Chuāndàhuáng* (川大黃 *Radix et Rhizoma Rhei Palmati*) and powder of *Huángbò* (黃檗 *Phellodendron amurense Rupr*), *1 qian* (3 g) and *1 zi* (0.45 g) respectively; *Qīngfěn* (輕粉 *Calomelas*) and *Náoshā* (硇砂 *Sal Ammoniac*), *5 fen* (1.5 g).

The ingredients mentioned above are ground into fine powder and mixed with flour dough to make pills as big as millet; the pills are taken with *Táozhītāng* (桃枝湯 *Decoction of Ramulus Persicae*). For each dose 5 to 7 pills are taken for children at the age of one year old; for children at the age of five to seven years old, *20* to *30* pills are taken with *Táozhītāng* (桃枝湯 *Decoction of Ramulus Persicae*); for children at the age of less than one year old, *2* or *3* pills are taken before bedtime.

058

Chánhuāsǎn

蟬花散

Powder of Cordyceps Cicadae

Chánhuāsǎn (蟬花散 *Powder of Cordyceps Cicadae*) is used to treat fright wind, night crying, teeth grinding and cough as well as swollen sore throat.

Chánhuā (蟬花 *Cordyceps Cicadae*) with its shell, straight *Báijiāngcán* (白僵蠶 *Bombyx Batryticatus*) stir-fried with wine and 甘草 (*Radix Glycyrrhizae Preparata*), *1 qian* (3 g) respectively; and *Yánhúsuǒ* (延胡索 *Rhizoma Corydalis*) *0.5 fen* (0.15 g).

The ingredients mentioned above are ground into powder; 1 *zi* (0.45 g) is taken for children at the age of one year old; *0.5 qian* (1.5 g) is taken for children at the age of four to five years old with *Chánkétāng* (蟬殼湯 *Decoction of Periostracum Cicadae*) after meal.

059

Gōuténgyǐnzǐ

鈎藤飲子

Drink of Ramulus Uncariae Rhynchophyllae cum Uncis

Gōuténgyǐnzǐ (鈎藤飲子 *Drink of Ramulus Uncariae Rhynchophyllae cum Uncis*) is used to treat vomiting and diarrhea due to deficiency of spleen and stomach and chronic fright with deficient wind.

Gōuténg (鈎藤 *Ramulus Uncariae Cum Uncis*) *3 fen* (0.9 g); *Chánké* (蟬殼 *Periostracum Cryptotympanae*), *Fángfēng* (防風 *Radix Saposhnikoviae*) deprived of root head and sliced, *Rénshēn* (人參 *Radix Ginseng*) deprived of root head and sliced, *Máhuáng* (麻黃 *Herbaephedrae Sinicae*) weighed after being deprived of joints, *Báijiāngcán* (白僵蠶 *Bombyx Batryticatus*) stir-fried to yellow, *Tiānmá* (天麻 *Rhizoma Gastrodiae*) and *Xiēwěi* (蠍尾 *Cauda Scorpionis*) deprived of toxin and stir-fried, *0.5 liang* (15 g); *Gāncǎo* (甘草 *Radix Glycyrrhizae Preparata*) and *Chuānxiōng* (川芎 *Rhizoma Chuanxiong*), *1 fen* (0.3 g) respectively; *Shèxiāng* (麝香 *Moschus*) *1 fen* (0.3 g) ground individually and mixed with other ingredients.

The ingredients mentioned above are ground into fine powder; for each dose *2 qian* (6 g) of the powder is decocted with a cup of water till water is left six in ten and then taken while the decoction is warm; the dosage is modified according to the age of child. For much cold involved, powder of *Fùzǐ* (附子*Radix Aconiti Lateralis Preparata*) *0.5 qian* (1.5 g) can be added and the decoction is taken anytime.

060

Bàolóngyuán(wan)

抱龍圓

Holding Dragon Pill

Bàolóngyuán (抱龍圓 *Holding Dragon Pill*) is used to treat coryza, epidemics, body heat, drowsiness, rough respiration, productive cough due to wind-heat and cold phlegm, convulsions due to fright-wind and periodic convulsions as well as insect poisoning and heatstroke. The pill can be taken after bath. Children with strong constitutions had better take it from time to time.

Tiānzhúhuáng (天竺黃 *Concretio Silicea Bambusae*) *1 liang* (30 g), *Xiónghuáng* (雄黃 Realgar) ground with water, *1 qian* (3 g); *Chénshā* (辰砂 *Cinnabaris*) and *Shèxiāng* (麝香 *Moschus*) ground individually, *0.5 liang* (15 g) respectively; *Tiānnánxīng* (天南星 *Rhizoma Arisaematis*) 4 *liang* (120 g), brewed in the ox gallbladder during the twelfth lunar month and then dried in the shade for 100 days; if there is no ox gallbladder, the raw *Tiānnánxīng* (天南星 *Rhizoma Arisaematis*) is peeled, dried and baked for application.

The ingredients mentioned above are ground into fine powder and mixed with boiled liquid of *Gāncǎo* (甘草 *Radix*

Glycyrrhizae) to make pills as big as *1 zaozi* (皂子 *Semen Gleditsiae Sinensis*); the pill can be taken after being dissolved in warm water. For children at the age of 100 days, *1* pill can be divided into three or four medications; *1* or *2* pills for children at the age of five years old; *3* to *5* pills for adults. It can also be used to treat leucorrhea of virgins. If the child is ill with latent summer-heat, *1* or *2* pills together with slight amount of salt can be chewed with fresh water. In the twelfth lunar month, the pill can be boiled with *Gāncǎo* (甘草 *Radix Glycyrrhizae*) and snow water, which has a better effect. Another method is as follows: *Tiānnánxīng* (天南星 *Rhizoma Arisaematis*) is steeped in malting water or fresh well water for three days; when being thoroughly soft, they are cooked for three or five times and taken out; immediately they are peeled and only the white and soft parts are selected to be sliced into thin pieces and dried by baking and stir-frying till yellow; *8 liang* (240 g) of the *Tiānnánxīng* powder is prepared. *Gāncǎo* (甘草 *Radix Glycyrrhizae*) *2.5 liang* (75 g) is beaten into fragments which are steeped in two bowls of water and cooked over a slow fire till half a bowl of water is left; after dregs of decoction are removed, the powder of *Tiānnánxīng* (天南星 *Rhizoma Arisaematis*) is sprinkled in and ground slowly till the liquid of *Gāncǎo* (甘草 *Radix Glycyrrhizae*) disappears; and then the other ingredients are put into it.

061

Dòujuànsǎn

豆卷散

Powder of Semen
Sojae Germinatum

Dòujuànsǎn (豆卷散 *Powder of Semen Sojae Germinatum*) is used to treat infantile chronic fright, usually due to overdose of medicine with much warmth or heat nature; thus the fright has not been relieved but the additional heat syndrome develops and in many cases the chronic fright may even turn into an acute one. The doctor should inquire into the medical history: How long has the disease lasted? Why does the patient get this disease? What medicine has the patient taken? This kind of disease can be relieved after giving some detoxifying agent with no exception and the formula proper is certainly effective.

Dàdòuhuángjuǎn (大豆黃卷 *Semen Sojae Germinatum*) refers to black beans that are steeped in water to sprout and then dried in the sun, *Bǎnlángēn* (板藍根 *Radix Isatidis*), *Guànzhòng* (貫眾 *Rhizoma Dryopteridis Crassirhizomatis*) and 甘草 (*Radix Glycyrrhizae Preparata*), *1 liang* (30 g) respectively.

The four ingredients mentioned above are ground into fine powder; for each dose *0.5–1 qian* (1.5–3 g) is decocted in water and taken after the dregs are removed. For the more severe case, the dosage can be increased to *3 qian* (9 g) and decoction with malting liquid with several drops of oil is recommended. The powder can also be used to treat vomiting with worms. It can be taken anytime.

062

Lóngnǎosǎn

龍腦散

Os Draconis Powder

Lóngnǎosǎn (龍腦散 *Os Draconis Powder*) is used to treat acute or chronic fright wind.

Dàhuáng (大黃 *Radix et Rhizoma Rhei Palmati*) steamed, *Bànxià* (半夏 *Rhizoma Pinelliae*) washed in hot water, cut into thin slices and steeped in ginger juice for one night, and then baked and stir-fried, *Gāncǎo* (甘草 *Radix Glycyrrhizae*), *Jīnxīngshí* (金星石 *Vermiculitum*), *Yǔyúliáng* (禹餘糧 *Limonitum*), *Bùhuīmù* (不灰木 *Asbesto*), *Qīnggéfěn* (青蛤粉 *Indigo Naturalis*), *Yínxīngshí* (銀星石 *Wavellite*) and *Hánshuǐshí* (寒水石 *Calcitum*).

The same amount of each of the ingredients mentioned above are ground into fine powder, which is ground additionally with *Lóngnǎo* (龍腦 *Borneolum Syntheticum*) *1 zi* (0.45 g) and stirred with fresh well water to *1 zi* (0.45 g) to *5 fen* (1.5 g) for medication; the dosage is modified according to the age of child and used to detoxify many kinds of toxins. The formula is an old one and is added by Dr. Qian Zhongyang with *2–3 twigs* of *Gānsōng* (甘松 *Radix et Rhizoma*

Nardostachyos), powder of *Huòxiāngyè* (藿香葉 *Herba Agastaches Rugosae*) *1 qian* (3 g), and *Jīnyáshí* (金牙石 *Vermiculitum*) *1 fen* (0.3 g) but the dosage of *Dàhuáng* (大黃 *Radix et Rhizoma Rhei Palmati*) is reduced by half; it has a wonderful effect treating medicinal intoxication and vomiting blood.

063

Zhìxūfēngfāng

治虛風方

Formula of Treating Deficient Wind

Zhìxūfēngfāng (治虛風方 *Formula of Treating Deficient Wind*) is used to treat vomiting and diarrhea of infants or deficient spleen leading to wind because of wrongly taking cold medicine for a long time which turns into chronic fright wind.

One *Tiānnánxīng* (天南星 *Rhizoma Arisaematis*) weighing over *8–9 qian* (24–27 g) is preferred.

Dig a pit about nine cm deep in the ground and make a fire with *five jin* (2.5 kilogram) of charcoal burnt to red; *Tiānnánxīng* (天南星 *RhizomaArisaematis*) is put into a container with half a cup of good wine over 2–3 charcoal; the pit is covered till *Tiānnánxīng* (天南星 *RhizomaArisaematis*) is slightly cracked which is then taken out to be filed into pieces; the pieces are then stir-fried evenly with no unripe part. After being cooled, *Tiānnánxīng* (天南星 *RhizomaArisaematis*) is ground into fine powder. For each dose *5 fen* (1.5 g) or *1 zi* (0.45 g) is taken or the dosage is modified according to the age of child. *Shēngjiāng* (生薑 *Rhizoma Zingiberis Recens*) and *Fángfēng* (防風 *Radix Saposhnikoviae*) are decocted densely for medication before meal or at any time.

064

Xūfēngyòufāng

虛風又方

Modified Formula of Treating Deficient Wind

Bànxià (半夏 *Rhizoma Pinelliae*) *1 qian* (3 g) washed in hot water for seven times, steeped with ginger juice for half a day and then dried in the sun; *Hòupò* (厚樸 *Cortex Magnoliae Officinalis*) from *Zǐzhōu 1 liang* (30 g) filed finely.

The ingredients mentioned above are steeped in three liters of rice washing water for 24 hours till the water disappears. If there is some water left at the 24th hour, the medicinals are boiled to dry and *Hòupò* (厚樸 *Cortex Magnoliae Officinalis*) is removed; only *Bànxià* (半夏 *Rhizoma Pinelliae*) is ground into fine powder. For each dose 0.5 or *1 zi* (0.225 or 0.45 g) is taken with mint decoction anytime.

065

Biǎnyínyuán(wán)

褊銀圓

Flat Mercury Pill

Biǎnyínyuán (褊銀圓 *Flat Mercury Pill*) is used to treat drooling due to wind, excessive Qi in diaphragm and heat in the upper region as well as indigestion of milk, abdominal distention and rough panting.

Bādòu (巴豆 *Fructus Crotonis*) deprived of rind, oil, core and membrane and ground into fine powder, and *Shuǐyín* (水銀 *Hydrargyrum*), *0.5 liang* (15 g) respectivly; *Hēiqiān* (黑鉛 *Graphite*) *2.5 qian* (7.5 g) is bound with *Shuǐyín* (水銀 *Hydrargyrum*) into granules; *Shèxiāng* (麝香 *Moschus*) *5 fen* (1.5 g) ground individually; good *Mò* (墨 *Inkstick*) *8 qian* (24 g) ground.

Fragments of *Bādòu* (巴豆 *Fructus Crotonis*) with good *Mò* (墨 *Inkstick*) are ground again evenly and then mixed with granules of *Hēiqiān* (黑鉛 *Graphite*), *Shèxiāng* (麝香 *Moschus*) and congee made of old rice to make pills as big as mung beans in flat shape; for children at the age of one year old, *1* pill is taken; 2 or 3 pills are recommended for children at the age of two or three years old and 5 or 6 pills for over five years old. The pills are taken with cooling decoction of mint after meal and the pills shouldn't be broken. The dosage can be modified according to the age.

066

Yòuniúhuánggāo

又牛黃膏

Modified Paste of Calculus Bovis

Yòuniúhuánggāo (又牛黃膏 *Modified Paste of Calculus Bovis*) is used to treat fright, fever due to coryza or due to infantile malnutrition and thirst concerned.

Xiónghuáng (雄黃 *Realgar*) ground, powder of *Gāncǎo* (甘草 *Radix Glycyrrhizae*) and *Chuāntiánxiāo* (川甜硝 *Natrii Sulfas*), *1 fen* (0.3 g) respectively; raw *Hánshuǐshí* (寒水石 *Calcitum*) ground with water, *1 liang* (30 g); powder of *Yùjīn* (郁金 *Radix Curcumae Wenyujin*) and *Nǎozi* (腦子 *Camphora*), *1 qian* (3 g) respectively; powder of *Lǜdòu* (綠豆 *Semen Vignae Radiatae*), *0.5 liang* (15 g).

The ingredients mentioned above are ground evenly into powder and mixed with refined honey to make paste; the paste as much as *0.5 zaozi* (皂子 *Semen Gleditsiae Sinensis*) is taken with decoction of mint after meal.

067

Wǔfú Huàdúdān

五福化毒丹

Toxin-Resolving Elixir with Five Blessings

Wǔfú Huàdúdān (五福化毒丹 *Toxin-Resolving Elixir with Five Blessings*) is used to treat remaining toxin of sore and rash surging up to mouth and teeth, leading to vexation and irritability, dry pharynx, sore in the mouth and tongue as well as to treat accumulative heat, toxic heat, fright and mania.

Shēngshú Dìhuáng (生熟地黃 *Radix Rehmanniae & Radix Rehmanniae Preparata*) baked and weighted, *5 liang* (150 g) respectively; *Yuánshēn* (元参 *Radix Scrophulariae*), *Tiānméndōng* (天門冬 *Radix Asparagi Cochinchinensis*) and *Màidōng* (麥門冬 *Radix Ophiopogonis Japonici*) deprived of core, baked and weighed, *3 liang* (90 g); *Zhìgāncǎo* (炙甘草 *Radix Glycyrrhizae Preparata*) and *Tiánxiāo* (甜硝 *Sweet Mirabilite*), *2 liang* (60 g) respectively; *Qīngdài* (青黛 *Indigo Naturalis*) *1.5 liang* (45 g).

The eight ingredients mentioned above are ground into fine powder and later ground again with *Tiánxiāo* (甜硝 *Sweet*

233

Mirabilite) and *Qīngdài* (青黛 *Indigo Naturalis*) additionally; the powder is mixed with refined honey to make pills as big as *Jītóu* (雞頭 (芡實) *Semen Euryales*); for each dose *0.5* or *1* pill is dissolved in water and taken after meal.

068

Qiānghuógāo

羌活膏

Paste of Rhizoma et Radix Notopterygii

Qiānghuógāo (羌活膏 *Paste of Rhizoma et Radix Notopterygii*) is used to treat deficiency of spleen and stomach, exuberant heat of liver Qi progressing to chronic fright, or chronic fright due to vomiting and diarrhea as well as to treat cold-damage.

Qiānghuó (羌活 *Rhizoma et Radix Notopterygii*) deprived of root head, *Chuānxiōng* (川芎 *Rhizoma Chuanxiong*), *Rénshēn* (人参 *Radix Ginseng*) deprived of root head, *Chìfúlíng* (赤茯苓 *Poria Rubra*) peeled, *Báifùzǐ* (白附子 *Rhizoma Typhonii Gigantei*) processed, *0.5 liang* (15 g) respectively; *Tiānmá* (天麻 *Rhizoma Gastrodiae*) *1 liang* (30 g), *Báijiāngcán* (白僵蠶 *Bombyx Batryticatus*) steeped in wine and fried to yellow, *Gānxiē* (幹蠍 *Scorpionis*) deprived of toxin, *Báihuāshé* (白花蛇 *Agkistrodon*) steeped in wine and its flesh baked to dry, *1 fen* (0.3 g), respectively; *Báifùzǐ* (白附子 *Radix Aconiti Lateralis Preparata*) processed and deprived of rind and nodes, *Fángfēng* (防風 *Radix Saposhnikoviae*) deprived of root head, sliced and baked, *Máhuáng* (麻黃 *Herbaephedrae Sinicae*) deprived of root head, sliced and baked and weighted after removing joints, *3 qian* (9 g) respectively; *Dòukòu* (豆蔻 肉 *Fructus Amomi Rotundus*), *Mǔdīngxiāng* (母丁香 *Fructus Syzygii Aromatici*), *Huòxiāngyè* (藿香葉 *Herba Agastaches Rugosae*), *Chénxiāng* (沉香 *Lignum Aquilariae Resinatum*) and *Mùxiāng* (木香 *Radix Aucklandiae*), *2 qian* (6 g), respectively; *Qīngfěn* (輕粉 *Calomelas*) *1 qian* (3 g), 珍珠 *Zhēnzhū* (珍珠 *Margarita*), *Shèxiāng* (麝香 *Moschus*) and *Niúhuáng* (牛黃 *Calculus Bovis*), *1 qian* (3 g) respectively; *Lóngnǎo* (龍腦 *Borneolum Syntheticum*) *0.5* zi (0.225 g); *Xiónghuáng* (雄黃 *Realgar*) and *Chénshā* (辰砂 *Cinnabaris*), *1 fen* (0.3 g) respectively; the seven ingredients mentioned above are ground respectively.

The ingredients mentioned above are ground into fine powder and mixed with boiled honey to make pills as big as soybeans; *1* to *2* pills are dissolved in warm decoction of mint or *Màidōng* (麥冬 *Radix Ophiopogonis Japonici*) and taken before meal. It is not suitable for cases with excessive heat and acute fright because of its warm nature. It can be taken anytime.

069

Yùlǐrényuán(wán)

鬱李仁圓

Pill of Semen Pruni Japonicae

Yùlǐrényuán (鬱李仁圓 *Pill of Semen Pruni Japonicae*) is used to treat infantile urinary and fecal retention due to febrile fright and phlegmatic excess, which needs to be purged.

Yùlǐrén (郁李仁 *Semen Pruni Japonicae*) peeled, and *Chuāndàhuáng* (川大黄 *Radix et Rhizoma Rhei Palmati*) deprived of rough rind to take the firm part, which is filed and steeped in wine for half a day, and the liquid is filtered out and then stir-fried into powders, *1 liang* (30 g) respectively; *Huáshí* (滑石 *Talcum*) 0.5 *liang* (15 g) ground finely.

Firstly *Yùlǐrén* (郁李仁 *Semen Pruni Japonicae*) is ground into paste and then mixed with *Dàhuáng* (大黄 *Radix et Rhizoma Rhei Palmati*) and *Huáshí* (滑石 *Talcum*) to make pills as big as millet; its dosage is modified according to the age of child and it is taken with milk or mint decoction before meal.

070

Xījiǎoyuán(wán)

犀角圓

Powder of Raw Rhinoceros Horn

Xījiǎoyuán (犀角圓 *Powder of Raw rhinoceros horn*) is used to treat febrile wind, excessive phlegm, red complexion, constipation and dysuria; as to heat evil in triple-Jiao and accumulation of toxin in viscera, it is an extremely reliable formula with the action of dispersion and purgation.

Fragments of raw *Xījiǎo* (犀角 *Cornu Rhinoceri Asiatici*) *1 fen* (0.3 g); *Rénshēn* (人参 *Radix Ginseng*) deprived of root head and sliced, *Zhǐshí* (枳實 *Fructus Aurantii Immaturus*) deprived of pulp and stir-fried with liquid adjuvant, *Bīngláng* (檳榔 *Semen Arecae*) *0.5 liang* (15 g) respectively; *Huánglián* (黃連 *Rhizoma Coptidis*) *1 liang* (30 g); *Dàhuáng* (大黃 *Radix et Rhizoma Rhei Palmati*) *2 liang* (60 g) steeped in wine and sliced; *100 Bādòu* (巴豆 *Fructus Crotonis*) peeled and stuck to *Dàhuáng* (大黃 *Radix et Rhizoma Rhei Palmati*) which is wrapped in paper and steamed in a rice pot for three times; the medicinal lump is cut into slices and stir-fried to brown with *Bādòu* (巴豆 *Fructus Crotonis*) being removed.

The ingredients mentioned above are ground into fine powder and mixed with refined honey to make pills as big as sesame seeds; for each dose, *10–20* pills are taken with boiled water before bedtime. If there is no effect, the number of pills can be increased. The pills are also used for adults and pregnant women without any harm.

071

Yìgōngsǎn
異功散
Extraordinary Merit Powder

Yìgōngsǎn (異功散 *Extraordinary Merit Powder*) has the action of warming the middle and harmonizing Qi and can treat vomiting and diarrhea and no appetite for milk. For the case with deficient cold disease, it can be taken first in several doses to invigorate Qi.

Rénshēn (人参 *Radix Ginseng*) deprived of root head, *Fúlíng* (茯苓 *Poria*) peeled, *Báizhú* (白術 *Rhizoma Atractylodis Macrocephalae*), *Chénpí* (陳皮 *Pericarpium Citri Reticulatae*) filed and *Gāncǎo* (甘草 *Radix Glycyrrhizae*), with the same dosage and stir-fried.

The ingredients mentioned above are ground into fine powder; for each dose, *2 qian* (6 g) of *Yìgōngsǎn* (異功散 *Extraordinary Merit Powder*) is decocted in a cup of water, with 5 pieces of *Shēngjiāng* (生薑 *Rhizoma Zingiberis Recens*) and 2 *Zǎo* (棗 *Fructus Jujubae*) till water is left seven in ten; the dedoction is taken before meal while it is warm and the dosage is modified according to the age.

072

Huòxiāngsǎn

藿香散

Powder of Herba Agastaches Rugosae

Huòxiāngsǎn (藿香散 *Powder of Herba Agastaches Rugosae*) is used to treat deficient heat of spleen and stomach, red complexion, vomiting with drooling, cough and obvious diarrhea.

Màidōng (麥門冬 *Radix Ophiopogonis Japonici*) deprived of core and baked, *Bànxià* (半夏 *Rhizoma Pinelliae*) stir-fried with malt, *Shígāo* (石膏 *Gypsum Fibrosum*) and *Gāncǎo* 甘草 (*Radix Glycyrrhizae Preparata*) stirred-fried with liquid adjuvent, *0.5 liang* (15 g) respectively; *Huòxiāngyè* (藿香葉 *Herba Agastaches Rugosae*) *1 liang* (30 g).

The ingredients mentioned above are ground into fine powder; for each dose *5 fen* to *1 qian* (1.5 to 3 g) of the powder in one and a half cups of water is decocted till water is left seven in ten and the medicine is taken with warm water before meal.

073

Rúshèngyuán(wán)

如聖圓

Saint-Like Pill

Rúshèngyuán (如聖圓 *Saint-Like Pill*) is used to treat diarrhea due to infantile malnutrition with alternative cold and heat.

Húhuánglián (胡黃連 *Rhizoma Picrorhizae*), *Báiwúyí* (白蕪荑 *Pasta Ulmi*) deprived of membranous wing and stir-fried and *Chuānhuánglián* (川黃連 *Rhizoma Coptidis*), *2 liang* (60 g) respectively; *Shǐjūnzǐ* (使君子 *Fructus Quisqualis*) *1 liang* (30 g) weighed after being deprived of shell; *Shèxiāng* (麝香 *Moschus*) ground individually, *5 fen* (1.5 g); *5* dry *Xiāmá* (蝦蟆 *Rana Siccus*) filed and boiled with wine to make paste.

The ingredients mentioned above are ground into powder and mixed with the paste to make pills as big as sesame seeds; for each dose, *5* to *7* pills for children at the age of two or three years old and *10* to *15* pills for children over three years old are taken with ginseng decoction anytime.

074

Báifùzǐ Xiāngliányuán(wán)

白附子香連圓

Pill of Rhizoma Typhonii Gigantei, Radix Aucklandiae and Rhizoma Coptidis

Báifùzǐ Xiāngliányuán (白附子香連圓 *Pill of Rhizoma Typhonii Gigantei, Radix Aucklandiae and Rhizoma Coptidis*) is used to treat Qi deficiency of stomach and intestine and drastic damage due to milk feeding with alternative cold and heat, diarrhea with bloody and mucous stool, tenesmus, abdominal cramp, frequent attacks and reduced ingestion of milk food.

Huánglián (黃連 *Rhizoma Coptidis*) and *Mùxiāng* (木香 *Radix Aucklandiae*) *1 fen* (0.3 g) respectively; two big *Báifùzǐ* (白附子 *Rhizoma Typhonii Gigantei*).

The ingredients mentioned above are ground into powder and mixed with cooked millet to make pills as big as mung beans or millet; for each dose *10* to *20–30* pills are taken with clear rice juice before meal, four or five times, during the day and at night respectively.

075

Dòukòu Xiāngliányuán(wan)

豆蔻香連圓

Pill of Semen Myristicae, Radix Aristolochiae and Rhizoma Coptidis

Dòukòu Xiāngliányuán (豆蔻香連圓 *Pill of Semen Myristicae, Radix Aristolochiae and Rhizoma Coptidis*) is used to treat diarrhea with bloody and mucous stool despite chill and fever, abdominal pain and even cramp with borborygmus due to disharmony of Yin and Yang; the pills can be applied to have magical effect.

Huánglián (黃連 *Rhizoma Coptidis*) stir-fried, *3 fen* (0.9 g); *Ròudòukòu* (肉豆蔻 *Semen Myristicae*) and *Nánmùxiāng* (南木香 *Radix Aristolochiae*), *1 fen* (0.3 g) respectively.

The ingredients mentioned above are ground into fine powder and mixed with cooked millet to make pills as big as rice grains; for each dose *10* to *20–30* pills are taken with rice juice before meal, four or five times, during the day and at night respectively.

076

Xiǎoxiāngliányuán(wán)

小香連圓

Small Pill of Radix Aucklandiae and Rhizoma Coptidis

Xiǎoxiāngliányuán (小香連圓 *Small Pill of Radix Aucklandiae and Rhizoma Coptidis*) is used to treat abdominal pain with alternative cold and heat, indigestion of water and grain and slippery diarrhea.

Mùxiāng (木香 *Radix Aucklandiae*) and *Hēzǐròu* (訶子肉 *Fructus Chebulae*) *1 fen* (0.3 g) respectively; *Huánglián* (黃連 *Rhizoma Coptidis*) *0.5 liang* (15 g) stir-fried.

The ingredients mentioned above are ground into fine powder and mixed with cooked rice to make pills as big as mung beans; for each dose *10* to *30–50* pills are frequently taken with rice juice before meal.

077

Èrshèngyuán

二聖圓

Two-Saint Pill

Èrshèngyuán (二聖圓 *Two-Saint Pill*) is used to treat infantile diarrhea on and off due to visceral disorders without being cured for long, leading to emaciation and even infantile malnutrition; it is better to take the pills routinely.

Chuānhuánglián (川黃連 *Rhizoma Coptidis*) deprived of root beard and *Huángbò* (黃檗 *Phellodendron amurense Rupr.*) deprived of rough rind, *1 liang* (30 g) respectively.

The ingredients mentioned above are ground into powder and put into *Zhūdǎn* (豬膽 *Fel Suillus*) that is boiled in water till the pig's gallbladder is ripe; then the powder of the ingredients are made into pills as big as mung beans; for each dose *20* to *30* pills are taken with rice juice anytime routinely and the dosage is modified according to the age.

078

Mòshízǐyuán(wán)

沒石子圓

Galla Turcica Pill

Mòshízǐyuán (沒石子圓 *Galla Turcica Pill*) is used to treat diarrhea, cloudy urine, infantile malnutrition, dysentery, slippery diarrhea and abdominal pain.

Mùxiāng (木香 *Radix Aucklandiae*) and *Huánglián* (黃連 *Rhizoma Coptidis*), *1 fen* (0.3 g) respectively; *1* piece of *Mòishízǐ* (沒石子 *Galla Turcica*); *3* pieces of *Dòukòu rén* (豆蔻仁 *Fructus Amomi Rotundus*) and *3* pieces of *Hēzǐròu* (訶子肉 *Fructus Chebulae*).

The ingredients mentioned above are ground into fine powder and mixed with cooked rice to make pills as big as sesame seeds; for each dose the pills are taken with rice juice before meal and the dosage is modified according to the age.

079

Dāngguīsǎn

當歸散

Powder of Radix Angelicae Sinensis

Dāngguīsǎn (當歸散 *Powder of Radix Angelicae Sinensis*) is used to treat chill without fever during thriving change.

Dāngguī (當歸 *Radix Angelicae Sinensis*) 2 *qian* (6 g); *Mùxiāng* (木香 *Radix Aucklandiae*), *Guāngùi* (官桂 *Cortex Cinnamomi Cassia*), *Gāncǎo* (甘草 *Radix Glycyrrhizae Preparata*), *Rénshēn* (人參 *Radix Ginseng*), 1 *qian* (3 g) respectively.

The ingredients mentioned above are pounded into pieces; for each dose 2 *qian* (6 g) of the powder is decocted with a cup of water till the water is left seven in ten with *3* pieces of *Shēngjiāng* (生薑 *Rhizoma Zingiberis Recens*) and *1 Zǎo* (棗 *Fructus Jujubae*) enucleated and then the decoction is taken.

080

Wēnbáiyuán(wán)

溫白圓

White-Warmed Pill

Wēnbáiyuán (溫白圓 *White-Warmed Pill*) is used to treat diarrhea, thin and weak body, infantile cold malnutrition and acute watery diarrhea due to deficiency and encumbrance of spleen Qi, as well as chronic fright leading to cold body and convulsions after vomiting and diarrhea or some chronic disease.

Raw *Tiānmá* (天麻 *Rhizoma Gastrodiae*) *0.5 liang* (15 g); *Báijiāngcán* (白僵蠶 *Bombyx Batryticatus*) processed, raw *Báifùzǐ* (白附子 *Rhizoma Typhonii Gigantei*), *Gānxiē* (幹蠍 *Scorpionis*) deprived of toxin and *Tiānnánxīng* (天南星 *RhizomaArisaematis*) filed, steeped in hot water for seven times and stir-fried to dry, *1 fen* (0.3 g) respectively.

The ingredients mentioned above are ground into powder, steeped in hot water and mixed with flour obtained during Cold Food Festival to make pills as big as mung beans; the pills are put into the flour for seven days and then taken out; *5–7* to *20–30* pills are taken with decoction of ginger and rice juice while fasting; the number of pills can be increased gradually and it is suitable to take the pills routinely as possible.

081

Dòukòusǎn

豆蔻散

Nutmeg Powder

Dòukòusǎn (豆蔻散 *Nutmeg Powder*) is used to treat vomiting, diarrhea, vexing thirst, abdominal distention and oliguria.

Dòukòu (豆蔻 *Fructus Amomi Rotundus*) and *Dīngxiāng* (丁香 *Flos SyzygiiAromatici*), *0.5 fen* (0.15 g) respectively; imported *Liúhuáng* (硫黃 *Sulfur*) *1 fen* (0.3 g); *Huáshí* (白滑石 *Talcum*) from *Guifu 3 fen* (0.9 g).

The ingredients mentioned above are ground into fine powder; for each dose *1 zi* to *0.5 qian* (0.45–1.5 g) is taken with rice juice anytime.

082

Wēnzhōngyuán(wán)

溫中圓

Middle-Warming Pill

Wēnzhōngyuán (溫中圓 *Middle-Warming Pill*) is used to treat stomach cold leading to diarrhea with indigestion of milk, abdominal pain, borborygmus, sour regurgitation, anorexia and acute and severe vomiting and diarrhea.

Rénshēn (人參 *Radix Ginseng*) deprived of root head and baked, *Gāncǎo* (甘草 *Radix Glycyrrhizae*) filed and baked, *Báizhú* (白術 *Rhizoma Atractylodis Macrocephalae*), *1 liang* (30 g) respectively, ground into powder.

The ingredients mentioned above are mixed with ginger juice and flour to make pills as big as mung beans and for each dose *10* to *20* pills are taken with rice juice at any time.

083

Húhuánglián Shèxiāngyuán(wán)

胡黄連麝香圓

Pill of Rhizoma Picrorhizae and Moschus

Húhuánglián Shèxiāngyuán (胡黄連麝香圓 *Pill of Rhizoma Picrorhizae and Moschus*) is a formula to treat evil Qi of infantile malnutrition, emaciation and white worms syndrome.

Húhuánglián (胡黄連 *Rhizoma Picrorhizae*) and *Báiwúyí* (白蕪荑 *Pasta Ulmi*) deprived of membranous wing, *1.5 liang* (45 g) respectively; *Mùxiāng* (木香 *Radix Aucklandiae*) and *Huánglián* (黄連 *Rhizoma Coptidis*), *0.5 liang* (15 g) respectively; *Chénshā* (辰砂 *Cinnabaris*) ground individually, *1 fen* (0.3 g); *Shèxiāng* (麝香 *Moschus*) filed and ground into powder, *1 qian* (3 g).

The ingredients mentioned above are ground into fine powder and mixed with flour to make pills as big as mung beans. For each dose *5–7* to *10* pills or *15* or *20* pills for children at the age of over 3–5 years old are taken with rice juice at any time.

084

Dàhúhuángliányuán(wán)
大胡黄連圓
Big Pill of Rhizoma Picrorhizae

Dàhúhuángliányuán (大胡黄連圓 *Big Pill of Rhizoma Picrorhizae*) can treat any manifestations of infantile fright malnutrition (involving heart), including abdominal distention, worm stirring, abnormal appetite for soil or raw rice, anorexia, drowsiness, constant crying, constipation or diarrhea due to visceral disorders, sallow skin and muscles and thin body, withering yellowish hair, thirst for water and vexing heat of five centers. It can kill worms, disperse distention, promote appetite, and treat sores and tinea; routine medication of the pill can prevent diarrhea.

Húhuánglián (胡黄連 *Rhizoma Picrorhizae*), *Huánglián* (黄連 *Rhizoma Coptidis*) and *Kǔliànzǐ* (苦楝子 *Fructus Melia Azedarach*), *1 liang* (30 g) respectively; *Báiwúyí* (白蕪荑 *Pasta Ulmi*) deprived of membranous wing, *0.5 lian* (15 g); *Lúhuì* (蘆薈 *Aloe*) collected in early autumn, *3 fen* (0.9 g) ground individually, and *Gānchántóu* (幹蟾頭 *Succys Bufo*), with preserved nature after being brunt, ground individually, *1 fen* (0.3 g) respectively; *Shèxiāng* (麝香 *Moschus*) *1 qian* (3 g),

253

ground individually; *Qīngdài* (青黛 *Indigo Naturalis*) *1.5 liang* (45 g), ground individually.

The first four ingredients mentioned above are ground into fine powder and mixed with pig gall to make pills as big as walnut; one piece of *Bādòurén* (巴豆仁 *Fructus Crotonis*) is put into *Zhūdǎnzhī* (豬膽汁 *Fel Suillus*) and wrapped in oil cloth to be steamed till ripe; then *Bādòurén* (巴豆仁 *Fructus Crotonis*) is removed and the ingredients are steamed with one liter of rice till ripe; finally they are mixed with the latter four ingredients to make pills. If it is hard to make pills, a little flour is added to make pills as big as sesame seeds; *10* to *20* pills are taken with rice juice, after meal or before sleep at *2–3* times a day.

085

Yúrényuán(wán)

榆仁圓

Pill of Siberian Elm Seed

Yúrényuán (榆仁圓 *Pill of Siberian Elm Seed*) is used to treat infantile malnutrition with heat syndrome, emaciation and worm syndrome; long-term medication can gather flesh.

Yúrén (榆仁 *Semen Ulmi Pumilae*) peeled, *Huánglián* (黃連 *Rhizoma Coptidis*) deprived of head, *1 liang* (30 g) respectively.

The ingredients mentioned above are ground into fine powder; then seven pig gall bladders are broken to take out the bile which is mixed with the powder of the two ingredients and steamed in a rice steamer for nine days, one time a day till the process is completed; *Shèxiāng* (麝香 *Moschus*) is ground into powder and *5 fen* (1.5 g) of the powder is steeped in hot water for a night and mixed with the powder and steamed cake to make pills as big as mung beans; for each dose *5–7* to *10–20* pills are taken with rice juice at any time.

086

Dàlúhuìyuán(wán)

大蘆薈圓

Big Aloe Pill

Dàlúhuìyuán (大蘆薈圓 *Big Aloe Pill*) is used to treat infantile malnutrition, kill worms, harmonize stomach and stop diarrhea.

Lúhuì (蘆薈 *Aloe*) ground into powder, *Mùxiāng* (木香 *Radix Aucklandiae*), *Qīngjúpí* (青橘皮 *PericarpiumCitri Reticulatae Viride*), *Húhuánglián* (胡黃連 *Rhizoma Picrorhizae*), *Huánglián* (黃連 *Rhizoma Coptidis*), *Báiwúyí* (白蕪荑 *Pasta Ulmi*) deprived of membranous wing and weighed, *Léiwán* (雷丸 *Omphalia*) broken (the white one is better, and the red one is lethal and is not allowed to be used.), *Hèshī* (鶴虱 *Fructus Carpesii*) slightly stir-fried, *0.5 liang* (15 g) respectively; *Shèxiāng* (麝香 *Moschus*) 2 *qian* (6 g) ground individually.

The ingredients mentioned above are ground into fine powder and mixed with cooked millet to make pills as big as mung beans, for each dose *20* pills are taken with rice juice at any time.

087

Lónggǔsǎn

龍骨散

Os Draconis Powder

Lónggǔsǎn (龍骨散 *Os Draconis Powder*) is used to treat infantile malnutrition, mouth sore and noma.

Pīshuāng (砒霜 *Arsenicum Sublimatum*) and *Chánsū* (蟾酥 *Venenum Bufonis*), *1 zi* (0.45 g) respectively; *Fěnshuāng* (粉霜 *Mercury Bichloride*) *5 fen* (1.5 g); *Lónggǔ* (龍骨 *Os Draconis*) *1 qian* (3 g); *Dìngfěn* (定粉 *Lead-Powder*) *1.5 qian* (4.5 g); *Lóngnǎo* (龍腦 *Borneolum Syntheticum*) *0.5 zi* (0.225 g).

Firstly *Pīshuāng* (砒霜 *Arsenicum Sublimatum*) is ground into extremely fine powder, then *Lónggǔ* (龍骨 *Os Draconis*) is added for grinding further and finally *Dìngfěn* (定粉 *Lead-Powder*) is added for grinding again; a small dosage of powder is applied on the focus each time.

088

Júliányuán(wán)

橘連圓

Pill of Pericarpium Citri Reticulatae and Rhizoma Coptidis

Júliányuán (橘連圓 *Pill of Pericarpium Citri Reticulatae and Rhizoma Coptidis*) is used to treat thin body due to infantile malnutrition, and long-term medication can help to digest food, harmonize Qi and grow in flesh.

Chénjúpí (陳橘皮 *Pericarpium Citri Reticulatae*) *1 liang* (30 g); *Huánglián* (黃連 *Rhizoma Coptidis*) *1.5 liang* (45 g) deprived of root beard and steeped in rice-washing water for one day.

The ingredients are ground into fine powder and *Shèxiāng* (麝香 *Moschus*) *5 fen* (1.5 g) is added to be ground again, which is put into the seven *Zhūdǎn* (豬膽汁 *Fel Suillus*) pig's gallbladders and cooked in *Jiāngshuǐ* (漿水 *Malting Liquid*); the gallbladders are pierced when they are becoming cooked; the gallbladders are taken out to make pills with millet porridge as big as mung beans. For each dose *10* to *20–30* pills are taken with rice juice anytime and the dosage is modified according to the age.

089

Lóngfěnyuán(wán)

龍粉圓

Pill of Radix Gentianae

Lóngfěnyuán (龍粉圓 *Pill of Radix Gentianae*) is used to treat thirst due to infantile malnutrition.

Cǎolóngdǎn (草龍膽 *Radix Gentianae*) and *Dìngfěn* (定粉 *Lead-Powder*) stir-fried slightly, *Wūméiròu* (烏梅肉 *Fructus Mume*) baked and weighed, *Huánglián* (黃連 *Rhizoma Coptidis*), *1 fen* (0.3 g) respectively.

The ingredients are ground into fine powder and mixed with refined honey to make pills as big as sesame seeds; *10* to *20* pills are taken with rice juice anytime.

090

Xiāngyínyuán(wán)

香銀圓

Hardness-Resolving Pill

Xiāngyínyuán (香銀圓 *Hardness-Resolving Pill*) is used to treat vomiting.

Dīngxiāng (丁香 *Flos Syzygii Aromatici*) and *Gāngě* (幹葛 *Radix Puerariae Thomsonii*), *1 liang* (30 g) respectively; *Bànxià* (半夏 *Rhizoma Pinelliae*) steeped in hot water for seven times, sliced and baked; *Shuǐyín* (水銀 *Hydrargyrum*), *0.5 liang* (15 g) respectively.

The first three ingredients mentioned above are ground into fine powder and *Shuǐyín* (水銀 *Hydrargyrum*) is added for grinding again which is mixed to make pills as big as sesame seeds. For each dose, *1–2* to *5–7* pills are taken anytime with the water boiled in a gold or silver container.

091

Jīnhuásǎn

金華散

Golden Luster Powder

Jīnhuásǎn (*Golden Luster Powder*) is used to treat dry or wet ulcer and tinea sore.

Huángdān (黃丹 *Minium*) calcined, *1 liang* (30 g); *Qīngfěn* (輕粉 *Calomelas*) *1 qian* (3 g); *Huángbò* (黃檗 *Phellodendron amurense Rupr.*) and *Huánglián* (黃連 *Rhizoma Coptidis*) *0.5 liang* (15 g) respectively, *and Shèxiāng* (麝香 *Moschus*) *1 zi* (0.45 g).

The ingredients mentioned above are ground into fine powder. Firstly, the sore surface is cleaned, and then the fine powder is put on it after the sore surface is dried. For dry tinea sore, the powder is mixed with lard oil in winter for application on the spot. Without lard oil, sesame oil can be used instead; *Huángqín* (黃芩 *Radix Scutellariae Baicalensis*) and *Dàhuáng* (大黃 *Radix et Rhizoma Rhei Palmati*) can be added.

092

Ānchóngyuán(wán)

安蟲圓

Parasite-Expelling Pill

Ānchóngyuán (安蟲圓 *Parasite-Expelling Pill*) is used to treat the deficiency of upper and middle Jiao, or to treat abdominal pain and roundworm disturbing due to cold in stomach. It is also called *Kǔliànyuánfāng* (苦棟圓方 *Chinaberry Root Pill*).

Gānqī (幹漆 *Resina Toxicodendri*) 3 *fen* (0.9 g) pounded into pieces and stir-fried till smoke disappears; *Xiónghuáng* (雄黃 *Realgar*) and *Bādòushuāng* (巴豆霜 *Semen Crotonis Pulveratum*) *1 qian* (3 g) respectively.

The ingredients mentioned above are ground into fine powder and mixed with flour to make pills as big as glutinous millet. The dosage is modified according to the age of the child. The pills are taken with the decoction of *Shíliúgēn* (石榴根 *Radix Granati Radicis*) which is grown towards the east. For abdominal pain, *five* or *seven* to *20–30* pills are taken with *Kǔliàngēntāng* (苦棟根湯 *Decoction of Chinaberry Root*) or *Wúyítāng* (蕪荑湯 *Decoction of Pasta Ulmi*) during attack.

093

Wúyísǎn

蕪荑散

Powder of Pasta Ulmi

Wúyísǎn (蕪荑散 *Powder of Pasta Ulmi*) is used to treat abdominal pain due to worm disease and stomach cold.

Báiwúyí (白蕪荑 *Pasta Ulmi*) deprived of membranous wring and weighed, and *Gānqī* (幹漆 *Resina Toxicodendri*) stir-fried, with the same dosage.

The ingredients mentioned above are ground into fine powder, and for each dose *1* zi (0.45 g), *5 fen* (1.5 g) or *1* qian (3 g) is dissolved in rice juice and taken during attack. The formula is the same as *Yangsheng Biyong Formula* (養生必用方) by Du Ren. Dr. Du's formula is also used to treat abdominal pain due to stomach cold.

094

Dǎnfányuán(wán)

膽礬圓

Chalcanthitum Pill

Dǎnfányuán (膽礬圓 *Chalcanthitum Pill*) is used to treat infantile malnutrition, dissipate the aggregation, improve appetite, stop diarrhea, harmonize stomach and expel worms.

Real *Dǎnfán* (膽礬 *Chalcanthitum*) *1 qian* (3 g), made into rough powder, real *Lǜfán* (綠礬 *Melanteritum*) *2 liang* (60 g), *14 big Zǎo* (棗 *Fructus Jujubae*) enucleated and good *Cù* (醋 *Vinegar*) *1 liter*.

The four ingredients mentioned above are decocted together till *jujube*s (*Zǎo* 棗 *Fructus Jujubae*) are tender and later they are mixed with the following ingredients.

Shǐjūnzǐ (使君子 *Fructus Quisqualis*) deprived of shell, *2 liang* (60 g); *Zhǐshí* (枳實 *Fructus Aurantii Immaturus*) deprived of shell and pulp and fried, *3 liang* (90 g); *Huánglián* (黃連 *Rhizoma Coptidis*) and *Hēlílè* (訶黎勒 *Fructus Chebulae*) enucleated, *1 liang* (30 g), respectively, and made into rough powder; *14 Bādòu* (巴豆 *Fructus Crotonis*) peeled and broken.

The five ingredients mentioned above are stir-fried together till black and dried until three in ten is left, which are mixed with the following ingredients.

Yèmíngshā (夜明砂 *Faeces Vespertilionis*) *1 liang* (30 g); ash of *Xiāmá* (蝦蟆 *Rana Siccus*), preserving its nature, *1 liang* (30 g); powder of *Kǔliàngēnpí* (苦楝根皮 *Cortex Meliae Azedarach*), 0.5 *liang* (15 g).

The three ingredients mentioned above are fried together till dried and are pounded together with the previous four ingredients into powder; then they are pounded 1000 times in mortar.

If a paste has not formed, more flesh of ripe *Dàzǎo* (大棗 *Fructus Jujubae*) *is* added; but it is not suitable to add too much, otherwise it is difficult to digest. If it is too viscous, warm water can be added in order to make pills as big as mung beans easily. For each dose *20* to *30* pills are taken together with rice juice or warm water anytime.

095

Zhēnzhūyuán(wán)

真珠圓

Pearl White Pill

Zhēnzhūyuán (真珠圓 *Pearl White Pill*) is used to get rid of any accumulation and aggregation, phlegm retention due to fright, food retention and breast lump and also to treat constipation, urinary retention, abdominal distention and to move stagnated Qi.

Mùxiāng (木香 *Radix Aucklandiae*), real *Báidīngxiāng* (白丁香 *Faeces Passeris*) and powder of *Dīngxiāng* (丁香 *Flos Syzygii Aromatici*), *0.5 qian* (1.5 g) respectively; *14* pieces of *Bādòu* (巴豆 *Fructus Crotonis*) steeped in water for one night and ground into fine powder, *Qīngfěn* (輕粉 *Calomelas*) *5 fen* (1.5 g), respectively, and a little of *Qīngfěn* (輕粉 *Calomelas*) left for coating; powder of *Huáshí* (白滑石 *Talcum*) *2 qian* (6 g).

The ingredients mentioned above are ground into powder, stirred evenly and burnt after being wrapped in wet paper, and finally mixed with cooked millet to make pills as big as sesame seeds. One pill for children at the age of one year old or *eight* pills for 8–9 to 15 years old, are decocted with processed *zaozi* (皂子 *Semen Gleditsiae Sinensis*) and taken after cooling. For the case complicated by febrile wind which is difficult to treat, a dose of cooling medicine is taken first; for the case with breast lump, the number of pills is reduced and the medicine is taken before bedtime every other day.

096

Xiāojiānyuán(wán)

消堅圓

Hardness-Resolving Pill

Xiāojiānyuán (消堅圓 *Hardness-Resolving Pill*) is used to eliminate breast lump, remove the harmful milk of feeding after intercourse and also treat phlegm due to heat evil and diaphragmatic excess and remove retention.

Powder of *Náoshā* (硇砂 *Sal Ammoniac*), *Bādòushuāng* (巴豆霜 *Semen Crotonis Pulveratum*) and *Qīngfěn* (輕粉 *Calomelas*), *1 qian* (3 g), respectively; the granules of *Shuǐyín* (水銀 *Hydrargyrum*) as much as *2 pieces of zaozi* (皂子 seed of *Chinese Honeylocust*), slight dosage of fine *Mò* (墨 *Inkstick*) and powder of *Huángmíngjiāo* (黃明膠 *Collacorii Bovis*) *5 qian* (15 g).

The ingredients mentioned above are ground together evenly into powder and mixed with flour to make pills as big as sesame seeds, which are taken with back-flowing water; *1* pill for children at the age of one year old is taken after meal.

097

Bǎibùyuán(wán)

百部圓

Radix Stemonae Pill

Bǎibùyuán (百部圓 *Radix Stemonae Pill*) is used to treat lung cold, productive cough and slight panting.

Bǎibù (百部 *Radix Stemonae*) stir-fried, *3 liang* (90 g), *Máhuáng* (麻黃 *Herbaephedrae Sinicae*) deprived of joints, *2 fen* (0.6 g) and *40* pieces of *Xìngrén* (杏仁 *Semen Armeniacae Amarum*) deprived of rind and spike, slightly stir-fried and boiled in water for three to five times.

The ingredients mentioned above are ground into powder and mixed with refined honey to make pills as big as *Qiànshí* (芡實 *Gordon Euryale Seed*) and *2* to *3* pills are taken after being dissolved in warm water anytime at three or four doses a day. This is an existing formula. Dr. Qian added *50 Sōngzǐ* (松子 *Pinus Pinea*) and mixed it with sugar to make pills, having wonderful effect if dissolved slowly in the mouth.

098

Zǐcǎosǎn

紫草散

Radix Lithospermi Pill

Zǐcǎosǎn (紫草散 *Radix Lithospermi Pill*) is used to promote eruption of macular rash.

Gōuténggōuzǐ (鉤藤鉤子 *Ramulus Uncariae Cum Uncis*) and *Zǐcǎoróng* (紫草茸 *Lacca*) with the same dosage.

The ingredients mentioned above are ground into fine powder; for each dose *1 zi* (0.45 g), *5 fen* (1.5 g) or *1 qian* (3 g) is dissolved in warm wine and taken anytime.

099

Qínjiāosăn

秦艽散

Powder of Radix Gentianae Macrophyllae

Qínjiāosăn (秦艽散 *Powder of Radix Gentianae Macrophyllae*) is a formula to treat tidal fiver, poor appetite and thin body during thriving change.

Qínjiāo (秦艽 *Radix Gentianae Macrophyllae*) deprived of root head, sliced and baked to dry; *Zhìgāncăo* (炙甘草 *Radix Glycyrrhizae Preparata*), *1 liang* (30 g), respectively; dry *Bòhe* (薄荷 *Herba Menthae Heplocalycis*) 0.5 liang (15 g), not baked.

The ingredients mentioned above are ground into rough powder; for each dose *1* to *2 qian* (3–6 g) of powder is decocted in a middle cup of water till the water is left eight in ten and taken while it is warm after meal.

100

Dìgǔpísǎn

地骨皮散

Cortex Lycii Radicis Powder

Dìgǔpísǎn (地骨皮散 *Cortex Lycii Radicis Powder*) is a formula to treat periodic deficient fever and also cold-damage with high fever or residual fever.

Dìgǔpí (地骨皮 *Cortex Lycii Radicis*), better if self-collected; *Zhīmǔ* (知母 *Rhizoma Anemarrhenae*); *Cháihú* (柴胡 *Radix Bupleuri Chinensis*) from Yinzhou and deprived of root head; *Gāncǎo* (甘草 *Radix Glycyrrhizae Preparata*); *Bànxià* (半夏 *Rhizoma Pinelliae*), washed in hot water for seven times, sliced and baked; *Rénshēn* (人參 *Radix Ginseng*) deprived of root head and baked; *Chìfúlíng* (赤茯苓 *Poria Rubra*), with the same dosage.

The ingredients mentioned above are ground into fine powder; for each dose 2 *qian* (6 g) of the powder is decocted with five pieces of *Shēngjiāng* (生薑 *Rhizoma Zingiberis Recens*) in a cup of water till the water is left eight in ten, and then taken while it is warm after meal; the dosage is modified according to the age of the child.

101

Rénshēn Shēngxīsǎn

人参生犀散

Powder of Ginseng and Raw Rhinoceros Horn

Rénshēn Shēngxīsǎn (人参生犀散 *Powder of Ginseng and Raw Rhinoceros Horn*) is used to disperse seasonal Qi causing infantile diseases, including cold congestion, cough, phlegm retention, panting and chest bloating, palpitation, fright and constipation or diarrhea due to visceral disorders as well as to improve appetite. It can also treat any febrile wind and diarrhea and poor appetite due to usual ingestion of cooling medicine.

Rénshēn (人参 *Radix Ginseng*) deprived of root head, *3 qian* (9 g); *Qiánhú* (前胡 *Radix Peucedani*) deprived of root head, *7 qian* (21 g); *Gāncǎo* (甘草 *Radix Glycyrrhizae Preparata*) stir-fried to yellow, *2 qian* (6 g); *Jiégěng* (桔梗 *Radix Platycodi*), *Xìngrén* (杏仁 *Semen Armeniacae Amarum*) deprived of rind and spike and slightly dried in the sun, made into powder and weighed, *5 qian* (15 g), respectively.

The ingredients mentioned above are ground into powder and later added with *Xìngrén* (杏仁 *Semen Armeniacae Amarum*), which are sifted through rough mesh; for each dose *2 qian* (6 g) is decocted with a cup of water till water is left eight in ten; after removing the dregs, the warm decoction is taken after meal.

102

Sānhuángyuán(wán)

三黄圓

Three-Yellow Pill

Sānhuángyuán (三黄圓 *Three-Yellow Pill*) is used to treat various kinds of fever.

Huángqín (黄芩 *Radix Scutellariae Baicalensis*) 0.5 liang (15 g) deprived of core; *Dàhuáng* (大黄 *Radix et Rhizoma Rhei Palmati*) peeled and roasted after being wrapped in wet paper, *Huánglián* (黄連 *Rhizoma Coptidis*) deprived of root beard, *1 qian* (3 g), respectively.

The ingredients mentioned above are ground into fine powder and mixed with flour to make pills as big as mung beans or sesame seeds; for each dose *5–7* to *15–20* pills are taken with rice juice after meal.

103

Tiānnánxīngsǎn

天南星散

Powder of Rhizoma Arisaematis Erubescentis

Tiānnánxīngsǎn (天南星散 *Powder of Rhizoma Arisaematis Erubescentis*) is used to treat failure of fontanel closure and stuffy nose.

Big *Tiānnánxīng* (天南星 *Rhizoma Arisaematis*) is selected to be processed and peeled, ground into fine powder and slightly stirred in vinegar and smeared on red silk fabric; then the fabric is applied on the spot that is warmed by the hand after the hand is warmed over the fire.

104

Huángqísǎn

黄芪散

Astragalus Powder

Huángqísǎn (黄芪散 *Astragalus Powder*) is used to treat deficient fever and night sweat.

Mǔlì (牡蠣 *Concha Ostreae*) calcined, *Huángqí* (黃芪 *Radix Astragali Mongolici*) and raw *Dìhuáng* (地黃 *Radix Rehmanniae*) with the same dosage.

The ingredients are ground into powder and decocted for medication at any time.

105

Hǔzhàngsǎn

虎杖散

Polygoni Cuspidati Powder

Hǔzhàngsǎn (虎杖散 *Polygoni Cuspidati Powder*) is used to treat excessive fever and night sweat.

Hǔzhàng (虎杖 *Rhizoma Polygoni Cuspidati*) is filed and decocted with water for medication at any time; the dosage is modified according to the age of the child.

106

Niǎntóusǎn

捻頭散

Twisting-Dough Powder

Niǎntóusǎn (捻頭散 *Twisting-Dough Powder*) is used to treat urine retention.

Yánhúsuǒ (延胡索 *Rhizoma Corydalis*) and *Chuānkǔliàn* (川苦楝 *Fructus Meliae Azedaarach*) with the same dosage.

The ingredients mentioned above are ground into fine powder; for each dose *5 fen* (1.5 g) or *1 qian* (3 g) of the powder is dissolved in decoction of twisting dough and the dosage is modified according to the age of the child. If there is no *Niǎntóutāng* (捻頭湯 *Twisting-Dough-Decoction*), several drops of oil can be added into the decoction and the medicine is taken before meal.

107

Yánggānsǎn

羊肝散

Goat Liver Powder

Yánggānsǎn (羊肝散 *Goat Liver Powder*) is used to treat sore and rash infiltrating eyes to form nebula.

The powder of *Chántuì* (蟬蛻 *Periostracum Cryptotympanae*), 2 or 3 *qian* (6 or 9 g), is dedocted in water with added *Yángzǐgāntāng* (羊子肝湯 *Decoction of Jecur Caprae*) and taken. Any pox is going to form crust, and the spot can be moistened with ghee or bran oil constantly; the scabs can be peeled immediately if possible; if the scabs are not moistened or peeled late, the crust will become hard and form scar insidiously.

108

Chántuìsǎn

蟬蛻散

Periostracum Cryptotympana Powder

Chántuìsǎn (蟬蛻散 *Periostracum Cryptotympana Powder*) is used to treat macular sore infiltrating eyes and is effective in one month for diseases with a history of not more than half a year.

Chántuì (蟬蛻 *Periostracum Cryptotympanae*) deprived of soil and pounded into powder, *1 liang* (30 g); *Zhūxuántíjiǎ* (豬懸蹄甲 *Pig Hoof Nail*) *2 liang* (60 g) put into a pot having the cover sealed with soil and salt, and burnt with preserving nature.

The two ingredients mentioned above are ground and stirred evenly after adding fine powder of *Língyángjiǎo* (羚羊角 *Cornu Saigae Tataricae*), *1 fen* (0.3 g); for each dose *1 zi* (0.45 g) or *5 fen* (1.5 g) for children at the age of 100 days and *1* to *2 qian* (3–6 g) for children at the age of over three years old is dissolved in warm water or fresh well water and taken after meal, three to four times during daytime and one to two times during the night. It is difficult to treat if the disease has a history of over one year.

281

109

Wūyàosǎn

烏藥散

Powder of Radix Linderae Aggregatae

Wūyàosǎn (烏藥散 *Powder of Radix Linderae Aggregatae*) is used to treat disharmony of cold and heat of lactating mother as well as abdominal pain sometimes or watery diarrhea or poor production of milk.

Wūyào (烏藥 *Radix Linderae Aggregatae*) from Tiantai, *Xiāngfùzǐ* (香附子 *Rhizoma Cyperi*) broken and white, *Gāoliángjiāng* (高良薑 *Rhizoma Alpiniae Officinarum*) and *Chìsháoyào* (赤芍藥 *Radix Paeoniae Rubra*).

The same amount of the ingredients mentioned above are ground into powder; for each dose *1 qian* (3 g) of powder is decocted with a cup of water till the water is left six in ten and taken with warm water. If there is heartache or abdominal pain the powder is decocted with wine; for watery diarrhea the powder is dissolved in rice juice and taken anytime.

110

Èrqìsǎn

二氣散

Two-Qi Powder

Èrqìsǎn (二氣散 *Two-Qi Powder*) is used to treat fright with alternative cold and heat evil leading to vomiting and nausea as well as various vomiting and diarrhea failing to be treated anyhow.

Liúhuáng (硫黃 *Sulfur*) 0.5 *liang* (15 g) ground into powder; *Shuǐyín* (水銀 *Hydrargyrum*) 2.5 *qian* (7.5 g), ground but with no crystal and with color like black coal.

One *zi* to five *fen* (0.45 to 1.5 g) of the medicinals mentioned above are taken after being dissolved in ginger decoction. Or they are stir-fried together to form granules into pills.

111

Tínglìyuán(wán)

葶藶圓

Papergrass Seed Pill

Tínglìyuán (葶藶圓 *Papergrass Seed Pill*) is used to treat feeding milk aspirated into lung leading to cough, red complexion and panting.

Tiántínglì (甜葶藶 *Semen Lepidii Apetali*) stir-fried wrapped in paper, *Hēiqiānniú* (黑牽牛 *Semen Pharbitidis*) stir-fried, *Hànfángjǐ* (漢防己 *Radix Stephaniae Tetrandrae*) and *Xìngrén* (杏仁 *Semen Armeniacae Amarum*) stir-fried and deprived of rind and spike, *1 qian* (3 g), respectively.

The ingredients mentioned above are ground into powder, added with *Xìngrénní* (杏仁泥 *Semen Armeniacae Amarum*), which is mixed with steamed old jujube flesh and pounded into pills as big as sesame seeds; for each dose 5 to 7 pills are taken with decoction of ginger.

112

Máhuángtāng

麻黃湯

Decoction of Chinese Ephedra Herb

Máhuángtāng (麻黃湯 *Decoction of Chinese Ephedra Herb*) is used to treat coryza, fever, no sweating, cough and panting.

Máhuáng (麻黃 *Herbaephedrae Sinicae*) deprived of joints, *3 qian* (9 g), cooked in water, filtered to remove foams and dried in the sun, and *Ròuguì* (肉桂 *Cortex Cinnamomi Cassiae*), *2 qian* (6 g); *Gāncǎo* 甘草 (*Radix Glycyrrhizae Preparata*), *1 qian* (3 g); seven *Xìngrén* (杏仁 *Semen Armeniacae Amarum*) deprived of rind and spike and sitr-fried with bran to yellow and ground into paste.

For each dose *1 qian* (3 g) is decocted in water and taken till sweating. It is not suitable for children with spontaneous sweating.

113

Shēngxī Mózhī

生犀磨汁

Wet-Grinding of Raw Rhinoceros Horn

Shēngxī Mózhī (生犀磨汁 *Wet-Grinding of Raw Rhinoceros Horn*) is used to treat difficult eruption of sore and rash, vomiting blood and nosebleeding.

Shēngxī (生犀 *Cornu Rhinoceri Asiatici*) ground with water into liquid.

The ingredient has an unspecified dosage and is ground into thick liquid in a container with rough interior wall using fresh well water. The liquid is slightly warmed and about a small cup is given to the child after milk feeding; its dosage is modified according to the age of the child.

114

Dàhuángyuán(wán)

大黃圓

Rhubarb Pill

Dàhuángyuán (大黃圓 *Rhubarb Pill*) is used to treat various kinds of febrile diseases.

Dàhuáng (大黃 *Radix et Rhizoma Rhei Palmati*) and *Huángqín* (黃芩 *Radix Scutellariae Baicalensis*), *1 liang* (30 g).

The ingredients mentioned above are ground into powder and mixed with refined honey to make pills as big as mung beans; for each dose *5* to *10* pills are taken with warm honey water and the dosage is modified according to the age of the child.

115

Shǐjūnzǐyuán(wán)

使君子圓

Fructus Quisqualis Pill

Shǐjūnzǐyuán (使君子圓 *Fructus Quisqualis Pill*) is used to treat visceral deficiency and incontinence of feces as well as infantile malnutrition with thin body, diarrhea, abdominal and hypochondriac distention and no appetite for milk; frequently taking the pills can relieve pain due to worm disease, benefit stomach, improve infantile malnutrition and gather flesh.

Hòupò (厚樸 *Cortex Magnoliae Officinalis*) deprived of rough rind and baked after smeared with ginger juice; *Gāncǎo* 甘草 (*Radix Glycyrrhizae Preparata*), *Hēzǐròu* (訶子肉 *Fructus Chebulae*) half raw and half ripe, and *Qīngdài* (青黛 *Indigo Naturalis*), *0.5 liang* (15 g), respectively; if the disease is complicated by fright or diarrhea due to heat evil, *Qīngdài* (青黛 *Indigo Naturalis*) can be added; if there is only infantile malnutrition with food retention and disharmony, *Qīngdài* (青黛 *Indigo Naturalis*) is not needed; *Chénpí* (陳皮 *Pericarpium Citri Reticulatae*) deprived of white pulp, *1 fen* (0.3 g); *Shǐjūnzǐ* (使君子 *Fructus Quisqualis*) deprived of shell, *1 liang* (30 g), cooked in a dough over a slow fire till cooked and the dough is discarded.

The ingredients mentioned above are ground into powder and mixed with refined honey to make pills the size of small *Jītóu* (芡實 *Semen Euryales*); for each dose *1* pill is taken with rice juice. For children at the age of from 100 days to one year old, *0.5* pill is taken after being dissolved in milk.

116

Qīngjīndān

青金丹

Bluish-Golden Elixir

Qīngjīndān (青金丹 *Bluish-Golden Elixir*) is used to disperse wind evil and promote expectoration.

Lúhuì (蘆薈 *Aloe*), *Yáxiāo* (牙硝 *Natrii Sulfas*) and *Qīngdài* (青黛 *Indigo Naturalis*) *1 qian* (3 g), respectively; 3 *Shǐjūnzǐ* (使君子 *Fructus Quisqualis*); *Péngshā* (硼砂 *Borax*) and *Qīngfěn* (輕粉 *Calomelas*) *5 fen* (1.5 g), respectively; *14* pieces of *Xiēshāo* (蠍梢 *Cauda Scorpionis*).

The ingredients mentioned above are ground into powder and stirred with ink liquid to make pills as big as sesame seeds; for each dose *3* pills are taken with decoction of mint.

117

Shāoqīngyuán(wán)

燒青圓

Bluish-Burning Pill

Shāoqīngyuán (燒青圓 *Bluish-Burning Pill*) is used to treat breast lump.

Qīngfěn (輕粉 *Calomelas*), *Fěnshuāng* (粉霜 *Mercury Bichloride*) and *Náoshā* (硇砂 *Sal Ammoniac*), *1 qian* (3 g) respectively; *Báimiàn* (白麵 *Flour*) *2 qian* (6 g); *Xuánjīngshí* (玄精石 *Selenitum*) *1 fen* (0.3 g), *Báidīngxiāng* (白丁香 *Faeces Passeris*) *1 zi* (0.45 g); *Dìngfěn* (定粉 *Lead-Powder*) *1 qian* (3 g); *Lóngnǎo* (龍腦 *Borneolum Syntheticum*) *0.5 zi* (0.225 g).

The ingredients mentioned above are ground into extremely fine powder and mixed with drops of water to make a cake which is cooked over a moderate fire till it is cooked but not charred; the cake is again ground into powder and mixed with drops of water to make pills as big as broom millet; for each dose 7 pills are taken with malting liquid. For children at the age of less than three years old, 5 pills are taken and the dosage is modified according to the age of children; it is an ancient formula.

118

Bàidúsǎn

敗毒散

Antiphlogistic Powder

Bàidúsǎn (敗毒散 *Antiphlogistic Powder*) is used to treat coryza, epidemic, rheumatism, dizziness, blurred vision, pain of four limbs, fearing cold, high fever, stiff nape and eye pain as well as chill, cough, stuffy nose and harsh voice.

Cháihú (柴胡 *Radix Bupleuri Chinensis*) washed and deprived of root head, *Qiánhú* (前胡 *Radix Peucedani*), *Chuānxiōng* (川芎 *Rhizoma Chuanxiong*), *Zhǐqiào* (枳殼 *Fructus Aurantii Submatures*), *Qiānghuó* (羌活 *Rhizoma et Radix Notopterygii*), *Dúhuó* (獨活 *Radix Angelicae Biserratae*), *Fúlíng* (茯苓 *Poria*), *Jiégěng* (桔梗 *Radix Platycodi*) stir-fried, and *Rénshēn* (人參 *Radix Ginseng*), *1 liang* (30 g) respectively; *Gāncǎo* (甘草 *Radix Glycyrrhizae*) 0.5 liang (15 g).

The ingredients mentioned above are ground into powder and *2 qian* (6 g) is taken each dose. If the powder is taken with the decoction of *Shēngjiāng* (生薑 *Rhizoma Zingiberis Recens*) and *Bòhé* (薄荷 *Herba Menthae Heplocalycis*), *Dìgǔpí* (地骨皮 *Cortex Lycii Radicis*) and *Tiānmá* (天麻 *Rhizoma Gastrodiae*) can be added. Or if the powder is chewed, *Chántuì*

(蟬蛻 *Periostracum Cryptotympanae*) and *Fángfēng* (防風 *Radix Saposhnikoviae*) can be added. In order to treat febrile fright, *Sháoyào* (芍藥 *Radix Paeoniae Alba*), *Gāngě* (幹葛 *Radix Puerariae Thomsonii*) and *Huángqín* (黃芩 *Radix Scutellariae Baicalensis*) can be added. If there is no sweating, *Máhuáng* (麻黃 *Herbaephedrae Sinicae*) can be added.

119

Mùguāyuán (Fùfāng)

木瓜圓 (附方)

Pill of Common Floweringqince Fruit (Appended)*

Mùguāyuán (木瓜圓 *Pill of Common Floweringqince Fruit*) is used to treat vomiting of newborn just after birth.

Powder of *Mùguā* (木瓜 *Fructus Chaenomelis Sprciosae*), *Shèxiāng* (麝香 *Moschus*), *Nìfěn* (膩粉 *Calomelas*), powder of *Mùxiāng* (木香 *Radix Aucklandiae*) and powder of *Bīngláng* (檳榔 *Semen Arecae*), *1 zi* (0.45 g), respectively.

The ingredients mentioned above are ground together into powder and mixed with flour to make pills as big as broom millet and for each dose *1* to *2* pills are taken with decoction of *Gāncǎo* (甘草 *Radix Glycyrrhizae*) anytime.

---

*This formula was not included in the original version of the book. It was added according to the Juzhen version.

120

Qīngjīndān (Fùfāng)
青金丹 (附方)
Bluish-Golden Elixir (Appended)*

Qīngdài (青黛 *Indigo Naturalis*) ground, *Xiónghuáng* (雄黃 *Realgar*) ground with water and *Húhuánglián* (胡黃連 *Rhizoma Picrorhizae*), *0.5 liang* (15 g), respectively; *Báifùzǐ* (白附子 *Rhizoma Typhonii Gigantei*) processed, *2 qian* (6 g), *Shuǐyín* (水銀 *Hydrargyrum*) *1 qian* (3 g), ground together with *Nìfěn* (膩粉 *Calomelas*); *Nìfěn* (膩粉 *Calomelas*) is ground together with *Shuǐyín* (水銀 *Hydrargyrum*), and added with *Xióngdǎn* (熊膽 *Fel Selenarcti*) dissolved in warm water; *Lúhuì* (蘆薈 *Aloe*) ground, and *Chánsū* (蟾酥 *Venenum Bufonis*) ground, *1 fen* (0.3 g) respectively. *Shèxiāng* (麝香 *Moschus*), *0.5 fen* (0.15 g), *Lóngnǎo* (龍腦 *Borneolum Syntheticum*)ground, *Zhūshā* (朱砂 *Cinnabaris*) ground with water and *Qiānshuāng* (鉛霜 *lead-cream*) ground, *1 zi* (0.45 g), respectively.

---

*This formula was not included in the original version of the book. It was added according to the Juzhen version.

The ingredients mentioned above are ground into fine powder and immersed in decocted *Zhūdǎnzhī* (豬膽汁 *Fel Suillus*) to mix with streamed cake to make pills as big as yellow millet. It is used to calm fright, treat wind, expel worms, relieve infantile malnutrition, get rid of various diseases, increase milk feeding, treat any kinds of fright wind and eyes turning up, convulsions of hands and feet and many other manifestations. One pill can be used and dissolved in warm water to drop into the nose and to make the child sneeze three to five times; additionally two pills can be used with mint decoction and the disease can be cured. For long-term infantile malnutrition of five kinds, abdominal distension, heavy head, thin and small limbs, pica of soil, anorexia for milk, biting nails, rubbing brows, sparse hair and varicose veins of the abdominal wall complicated by diarrhea, two pills can be taken with rice juice. For red ulceration in the lower part of the nose, worms in mouth and teeth due to infantile malnutrition and mouth sore, two pills can be ground with milk and applied on the affected part. For malnutrition involving eyes and night blindness, one lump of liver of white sheep is opened with a bamboo knife with two pills put inside, and sealed with twine to be steamed with rice-washed water; then the child can take it while fasting. The nursing mother should avoid fish, garlic, chicken, duck and pork. If one dose of the pill is taken every two to three days, the child will have no diseases forever and can avoid an early death. This is an ancient formula and Dr. Qian only doubles the dose of *Shèxiāng* (麝香 *Moschus*).

121

Shēngxīsăn (Fùfāng)

生犀散 (附方)

Raw Rhinoceros Horn Powder (Appended)*

Shēngxīsăn (生犀散 *Raw Rhinoceros Horn Powder*) is used to remove toxic Qi and relieve internal heat.

If raw *Shēngxī* (生犀 *Cornu Rhinoceri Asiatici*) is used, any containers that have been steamed or cooked are not allowed to be used and a new cooker is preferred.

Shēngxī (生犀 *Cornu Rhinoceri Asiatici*) of varied dosage is put into the container with rough interior wall and ground with fresh well water into thick liquid which is taken with a cup of warm tea after milk feeding; its dosage is modified according to the age of the child.

---

*This formula was not included in the original version of the book. It was added according to the Juzhen version.

122

Dàhuángyuán(wán) (Fùfāng)

大黃圓 (附方)

Rhubarb Pill (Appended)*

Dàhuángyuán (大黃圓 *Rhubarb Pill*) is used to treat febrile wind with internal excess, hot breath from mouth, constipation, dark urine, constant thirst for water and any syndrome to be treated with purging.

Chuānxiōng (川芎 *Rhizoma Chuanxiong*) *0.5 liang* (15 g) filed; *Hēiqiānniú* (黑牽牛 *Semen Pharbitidis*) *0.5 liang* (15 g) stir-fried to half cooked; *Dàhuáng* (大黃 *Radix et Rhizoma Rhei Palmati*) *1 liang* (30 g) washed with wine, steamed with rice and then cut into pieces for drying in the burning sun; *Gāncǎo* (甘草 *Radix Glycyrrhizae*) *1 fen* (0.3 g) filed and stir-fried with adjuvant.

The ingredients mentioned above are ground into fine powder and mixed with thin dough to make pills as big as sesame seeds; for each dose *10* pills for children at the age of two

---

*This formula was not included in the original version of the book. It was added according to the Juzhen version.

298

years old are taken with warm honey water after milk feeding till diarrhea develops; if there is no diarrhea, the number of pills can be increased for medication and the dosage is modified according to the condition of deficiency or excess.

123

Zhènxīnyuán(wán) (Fùfāng)

鎮心圓 (附方)

Heart-Settling Pill (Appended)*

Zhènxīnyuán (鎮心圓 *Heart-Settling Pill*) is used to cool heart meridian and treat febrile fright and profuse phlegm.

White *Tiánxiāo* (甜硝 *Sweet Mirabilite*), *Rénshēn* (人參 *Radix Ginseng*) deprived of root head and ground into powder, *Gāncǎo* 甘草 (*Radix Glycyrrhizae Preparata*) ground into powder and *Hánshuǐshí* (寒水石 *Calcitum*) burnt, *1 liang* (30 g) respectively; white and dry *Shānyào* (山藥 *Rhizoma Dioscoreae Oppositae*) and *Báifúlíng* (白茯苓 *Poria*), *2 liang* (60 g), respectively; *Zhūshā* (硃砂 *Cinnabaris*) *1 liang* (30 g), *Lóngnǎo* (龍腦 *Borneolum Syntheticum*) and *Shèxiāng* (麝香 *Moschus*), *1 qian* (3 g), respectively; the last three ingredients are ground into powder.

The ingredients mentioned above are ground into powder and mixed with ripe honey to make pills as big as *Qiànshí*

---

*This formula was not included in the original version of the book. It was added according to the Juzhen version.

(芡實 *Semen Euryales*). In order to make pills red, *2 qian* (6 g) of *Pīzǐyānzhī* (坯子胭脂 *Dactylopius Coccus Costa*) is added, that is, applying rouge color to pills. *Half a* pill to *1–2* pills are dissolved in warm water and taken after meal.

124

Liángjīngyuán(wán) (Fùfāng)

涼驚圓 (附方)

Fright-Cooling Pill (Appended)*

Péngshā (硼砂 *Borax*) ground, *Fěnshuāng* (粉霜 *Mercury Bichloride*) ground into powder, *Yùlǐrén* (郁李仁 *Semen Pruni Japonicae*) peeled, baked to dry and ground into powder, *Qīngfěn* (輕粉 *Calomelas*), *Tiěfěn* (鐵粉 *Ferrous Pulveres*) ground into powder, powder of *Báiqiānniú* (白牽牛 *Semen Pharbitidis*), *1 qian* (3 g) respectively; good *Làchá* (臘茶 *winter-tea*) *3 qian* (9 g).

The ingredients mentioned above are ground into fine powder and boiled with pear into paste to make pills as big as mung beans. *One to 3* pills are dissolved in water containing *Lóngnǎo* (龍腦 *Borneolum Syntheticum*) and taken after meal. It is also called *Lízhī Bǐngzǐ* (梨汁餅子 *Cake of Pear Juice*). The pills are also used to treat wind drooling of adult.

---

*This formula was not included in the original version of the book. It was added according to the Juzhen version.

125

Dúhuóyǐnzǐ (Fùfāng)

獨活飲子 (附方)

Angelicae Pubescentis Liquid (Appended)*

Dúhuóyǐnzǐ (獨活飲子 *Angelicae Pubescentis Liquid*) is a good formula to treat infantile malnutrition associated with kidney with fetid breath.

Tiānmá (天麻 *Rhizoma Gastrodiae*), *Mùxiāng* (木香 *Radix Aucklandiae*), *Dúhuó* (獨活 *Radix Angelicae Biserratae*) and *Fángfēng* (防風 *Radix Saposhnikoviae*), *1 qian* (3 g), respectively; *Shèxiāng* (麝香 *Moschus*) a little amount, mixed and ground into powder.

One qianbi (1.8 g) of the powder or *0.5 qian* (1.5 g) for younger children is taken with boiled decoction of *Màidōng* (麥門冬 *Radix Ophiopogonis Japonici*).

---

*This formula was not included in the original version of the book. It was added according to the Juzhen version.

126

Sānhuángsǎn (Fùfāng)

三黃散 (附方)

Three-Yellow Powder (Appended)*

Sānhuángsǎn (三黃散 *Three-Yellow Powder*) is a good formula to treat infantile malnutrition associated with kidney with tooth breakdown.

Niúhuáng (牛黃 *Calculus Bovis*), *Dàhuáng* (大黃 *Radix et Rhizoma Rhei Palmati*), *Shēngdìhuáng* (生地黃 *Radix Rehmanniae*), *Mùxiāng* (木香 *Radix Aucklandiae*) and *Qīngdài* (青黛 *Indigo Naturalis*) with the same amount, ground into powder.

One qianbi (1.8 g) of the powder is taken with boiled water for each dose.

---

*This formula was not included in the original version of the book. It was added according to the Juzhen version.

127

Rénshēnsǎn (Fùfāng)

人参散 (附方)

Ginseng Powder (Appended)*

Rénshēnsǎn (人参散 *Ginseng Powder*) is a good formula to treat infantile malnutrition associated with kidney with ulcerative alveolus.

Ròudòukòu (肉豆蔻 *Semen Myristicae*) processed, *Húhuánglián* (胡黄连 *Rhizoma Picrorhizae*), *Rénshēn* (人参 *Radix Ginseng*), *Xìngrén* (杏仁 *Semen Armeniacae Amarum*) stir-fried and *Zhìgāncǎo* (炙甘草 *Radix Glycyrrhizae Preparata*) with the same amount and ground into powder.

One qianbi (1.8 g) of the powder or *0.5 qian* (1.5 g) for younger children is taken with warm boiled water.

---

*This formula was not included in the original version of the book. It was added according to the Juzhen version.

128

Bīnlángsǎn (Fùfāng)
檳榔散 (附方)
Areca Powder (Appended)*

Bīnlángsǎn (檳榔散 *Areca Powder*) is used to treat infantile malnutrition associated with kidney with gum bleeding.

Mùxiāng (木香 *Radix Aucklandiae*), *Bīngláng* (檳榔 *Semen Arecae*), *Rénshēn* (人參 *Radix Ginseng*), *Huánglián* (黄連 *Rhizoma Coptidis*), *Zhìgāncǎo* (炙甘草 *Radix Glycyrrhizae Preparata*), with the same amount and ground into powder.

For each dose *1 qian* (3 g) of the powder or *0.5 qian* (1.5 g) for younger children is taken with boiled water.

---

*This formula was not included in the original version of the book. It was added according to the Juzhen version.

129

Huángqísǎn (Fùfāng)

黄芪散 (附方)

Astragalus Powder (Appended)*

Huángqísǎn (黃芪散 *Astragalus Powder*) is used treat infantile malnutrition involving kidney and rotten root.

Huángqín (黃芩 *Radix Scutellariae Baicalensis*) stir-fried with honey, *Niúhuáng* (牛黃 *Calculus Bovis*), *Rénshēn* (人參 *Radix Ginseng*), *Tiānmá* (天麻 *Rhizoma Gastrodiae*), *Xiē* (蠍 *Scorpio*) deprived of toxin, *Xìngrén* (杏仁 *Semen Armeniacae Amarum*) stir-fried, *Báifúlíng* (白茯苓 *Poria*), *Chuāndāngguī* (川當歸 *Radix Angelicae Sinensis*), raw *Dìhuán* (地黃 *Radix Rehmanniae*) washed and *Shúgān Dìhuáng* (熟幹 地黃 *Radix Rehmanniae Preparata*) washed, with the same amount and ground into powder.

For each dose *0.5 Qianbi* (0.9 g) for younger children is taken with decoction of *Tiānméndōng* (天門冬 *Radix Asparagi Cochinchinensis*) or *Màiméndōng* (麥門冬 *Radix Ophiopogonis Japonici*).

---

*This formula was not included in the original version of the book. It was added according to the Juzhen version.

130

Dìgǔpísǎn (Fùfāng)

地骨皮散 (附方)

Cortex Lycii Radicis Powder
(Appended)*

Dìgǔpísǎn (地骨皮散 *Cortex Lycii Radicis Powder*) is a good formula to treat infantile malnutrition associated with kidney with ulceration of gingiva and palate and the oral fetid odor or frequent bleeding.

Raw and dry *Dìhuáng* (地黄 *Radix Rehmanniae*) 0.5 *liang* (15 g), real *Dìgǔpí* (地骨皮 *Cortex Lycii Radicis*) and *Xìxīn* (細辛 *Herba Asari Manchurici*) 1 *fen* (0.3 g) respectively, *Wǔbèizǐ* (五倍子 *Galla Chinensis*) stir-fried to brown, 2 *qian* (6 g).

The ingredients mentioned above are made into powder and a small dosage is applied each time; it is just well to apply it frequently because of its therapeutic effect. It is commented that, according to the classical record, there are five kinds of

---

*This formula was not included in the original version of the book. It was added according to the Juzhen version.

infantile malnutrition which are associated with five viscera and are so named. Now the infantile malnutrition associated with only kidney has five manifestations and more importantly it is quite different from the common type, that is, gingival malnutrition. This disease has five stages according to its severity and can progress so quickly and dreadfully that the disease is otherwise known as noma "running horse" which is not an exaggeration. At the onset, the child has fetid odor and dry opening of stomach, depressing foul breath; later the disease progresses to damage sinews and the child has gingival sore, swelling or ulceration, and blackening teeth; progressing further, there appear sore, pustules and purulent ulceration in alveoli; being worse in progress, the heat evil is forced into vessels to cause bleeding and if its heat lingers for long, the gum will become rotten, alveoli widened and teeth lost; if the child lost all the teeth at the age of 6–7 years old, he cannot survive and can the disease be incurable? Now the wonderful formula is provided which should be given immediately as soon as there develops the disease and adjusted according to its changes of severity before the disease worsens.

131

Lánxiāngsǎn (Fùfāng)

蘭香散 (附方)

Herba seu Radix Caryopteridis Incanae Powder (Appended)*

Lánxiāngsǎn (蘭香散 *Herba seu Radix Caryopteridis Incanae Powder*) is used to treat noma with rotten teeth and even tooth breakdown, gum bleeding and tooth loss.

Qīngfěn (輕粉 *Calomelas*) and powder of *Lánxiāng* (蘭香 *Herba seu Radix Caryopteridis Incanae*), *1 qian* (3 g), respectively; *Mìtuósēng* (密陀僧 *Lithargyrum*) 0.5 *liang* (15 g) quenched in vinegar and ground into powder.

The ingredients mentioned above are ground into powder which is applied on the diseased teeth and gum with instant effect. The comment is that, if the infant is ill, the manifestations are mostly concerned with infantile malnutrition due to depressed Qi in triple-Jiao. Infantile malnutrition has five classifications based on five viscera. Among them the one is

---

*This formula was not included in the original version of the book. It was added according to the Juzhen version.

associated with kidney and is generally caused by kidney deficiency termed acute infantile malnutrition and its condition changes rapidly like a running horse, which is rather difficult to treat. The progress of the disease can be classified as follows: at the onset there appears fetid breath termed halitosis; secondarily there appears black tooth termed tooth breakdown; then there appears rotten gum termed ulcerative alveolus; at further stage there appears bleeding termed gum bleeding; at rampant stage the tooth is spontaneously lost termed rotten root. Since the tooth root is decayed, why does it need to be treated? Oh! To raise their children, the rich families tend to feed them with sweet and greasy food so that the children's kidney is easily affected by deficient heat or the women during pregnancy are addicted to greasy food so that the offspring are affected, which is not an occasional outcome. Now the secret formula is revealed in the text that follows.

132

Chuánchǐ Lìxiàosǎn (Fùfāng)

傳齒立效散 (附方)

Instant Powder for
Teeth Disease due to Infantile
Malnutrition (Appended)*

Yāzuǐdǎnfán (鴨嘴膽礬 *Chalcanthitum*) *1 qianbi* (1.8 g), roasted and ground with slight amount of *Shèxiāng* (麝香 *Moschus*).

The ingredients mentioned above are ground evenly and a small dosage is put onto the roots of teeth. In another formula *Chánsū* (蟾酥 *Venenum Bufonis*) *1 zi* (0.45 g) is mixed evenly with *Shèxiāng* (麝香 *Moschus*) for application. It is commented that the flowing of blood embodies nutrition while the circulation of Qi embodies defense. If there is damage to the nutrition and defense after full thriving change or during feeding, it is probable to cause various diseases. Maybe there appears Qi damage due to toxin and blood damage due to heat

---

* This formula was not included in the original version of the book. It was added according to the Juzhen version.

312

and where toxic heat attacks, the deficient viscus is easy to be affected; which viscus affected is in the most deficient status? The infantile kidney is often in the deficient status and shouldn't be attacked by toxic heat which involves sinews and bones; only teeth receive the remaining Qi of bone, so the teeth develop relative diseases first; it progresses as quickly as a running horse (noma), which has nothing to do with gradual development in fact. The suitable medicine includes *Gānlùyǐn* (甘露飲 *Sweet Dew Liquid*), *Dìhuánggāo* (地黄膏 *Six-Ingredient Rehmannia Paste*), *Huàdúdān* (化毒丹 *Toxin-Resolving Elixir*) and *Xiāodúyǐn* (消毒飲 *Toxin-Dispersed Liquid*). The treatment for the external syndrome includes the application of *Lìxiàosǎn* (立效散 *Instant-Effective Powder*) and *Shèchángāo* (麝酥膏 *Paste of Moschus and Venenum Bufonis*) and toxic heat-containing food should be avoided. This infantile malnutrition is different from the common syndromes and the first medical goal is to save the life of the patient. It is difficult to cure the disease with the common formulas.

133

Kēbǒyuán(wán) (Fùfāng)
蚵皮圓 (附方)
Toad Pill (Appended)*

Kēbǒyuán (蚵皮 *Toad Pill*) is used to treat five kinds of infantile malnutrition, eight types of diarrhea, improper milk feeding and abnormal temperature regulation; dry yellow hair, withered skin, thin legs with bulging abdomen, delayed closure of fontanels, sternal depression and gradual emaciation; frequent fever, night sweat, cough, swollen node on the back of the head, mass in the abdomen and cloudy urine like rice-washing water; diarrhea with pus and blue feces, rubbing eyebrows, nail biting, ingestion of soil, addiction to sweet and sour food, vomiting and indigestion; frequent vexation and thirst, poor awareness, red nose and dry lips; small worms coming out and heartache due to roundworm, keratomalacia and night blindness, termed *Dīngxīgān* (丁奚疳 infantile malnutrition due to excessive feeding). The medicinal pill has magic effect for this disease.

---

*This formula was not included in the original version of the book. It was added according to the Juzhen version.

Kēbǒ (蚵皮 *Succy Bufo*) immersed in wine, deprived of bone and baked, *Báiwúyí* (白蕪荑 *Pasta Ulmi*) deprived of rind, *Huánglián* (黃連 *Rhizoma Coptidis*) deprived of root beard, *Húhuánglián* (胡黃連 *Rhizoma Picrorhizae*) *1.5 liang* (45 g), respectively; *Qīngdài* (青黛 *Indigo Naturalis*) *0.5 liang* (15 g) as pill coating.

The ingredients mentioned above are ground into fine powder and mixed with pig bile and flour to make pills as big as millet; for each dose *30* pills are taken with rice juice after meal or before bedtime, three times a day.

Appendix: Translation of TCM Medicinals

Simplified Chinese	Pin Yin/Traditional Chinese/Latin Name	Common Name	Zheng Ming Ci Dian Dictionary
阿胶	Ējiāo (阿膠 *Colla Corii Asini*)	*Ass-Hide Gelatin*	10.212
巴豆	Bādòu (巴豆 *Fructus Crotonis*)	*Purging Croton Seed*	6.184
巴豆霜	Bādòushuāng (巴豆霜 *Semen Crotonis Pulveratum*)	*Defatted Croton Seed Powder*	9.36
白丁香, 麻雀粪	Baidingxiang (白丁香 *Faeces Passeris*)	*Sparrow Faeces*	10.161
白矾	Báifán (白礬 *Alumen*)	*Alum*	11.24
白茯苓, 茯苓	Báifúlíng (白茯苓 *Poria*)	*Tuckahoe*	8.42
白附子	Báifùzǐ (白附子 *Rhizoma Typhonii Gigantei*)	*Giant Typhonium Tuber*	1.1659
白甘遂	Báigānsuí (白甘遂 *Radix Kansui*)	*Kansui Root*	1.397
白花蛇	Báihuāshé (白花蛇 *Agkistrodon*)	*Long-Nosed Pit Viper*	10.155

白及	*Báijí* (白及 *Rhizoma Bletillae Striatae*)	*Common Bletilla Tuber*	1.1951
白僵蚕	*Báijiāngcán* (白僵蠶 *Bombyx Batryticatus*)	*Stiff Silkworm*	10.53
白面	*Báimiàn* (白麵 *Flour*)	*Flour*	
白芍,芍药	*Báisháo* (白芍 *Radix Paeoniae Alba*)	*White Peony Root*	1.746
白术	*Báizhú* (白術 *Rhizoma Atractylodis Macrocephalae*)	*Largehead Atractylodes Rhizome*	1.867
白土, 白垩	*Báitǔ* (白土, 白堊 *Calcium Carbonate*)	*Chalk*	
白芜荑	*Báiwúyí* (白蕪荑 *Pasta Ulmi*)	*Bigfruit Elm Pasdt*	9.33
百部	*Bǎibù* (百部 *Radix Stemonae*)	*Sessile Stemona Root Tuber*	1.1608
板蓝根	*Bǎnlángēn* (板藍根 *Radix Isatidis*)	*Isatis Root*	1.1180
半夏	*Bànxià* (半夏 *Rhizoma Pinelliae*)	*Pinellia Rhizome*	1.1612
半夏, 生半夏	*Shēngbànxià* (半夏 *Rhizoma Pinelliae*)	*Ternate Pinellia*	1.1612

(*Continued*)

(Continued)

Simplified Chinese	Pin Yin/Traditional Chinese/Latin Name	Common Name	Zheng Ming Ci Dian Dictionary
半夏曲	*Bànxiàqū* (半夏曲 *Rhizoma Pinelliae Fermentata*)	*Fermented Pinellia*	1.1612
薄荷	*Báohé* (薄荷 *Herba Menthae Heplocalycis*)	*Wild Mint Herb*	7.776
鳖甲	*Biējiǎ* (鱉甲 *Carapax Trionycis*)	*Turtle Carapace*	10.103
槟榔	*Bīngláng* (檳榔 *Semen Arecae*)	*Betelnutpalm Seed*	6.616
不灰木	*Búhuīmù* (不灰木 *Asbesto*)	*Asbestos*	11.64
草龙胆, 龙胆	*Cǎolóngdǎn* (草龍膽 *Radix Gentianae*)	*Chinese Gentian Root*	1.428
柴胡	*Cháihú* (柴胡 *Radix Bupleuri Chinensis*)	*Chinese Thorowax Root*	1.100
蝉花	*Chánhuā* (蟬花 *Cordyceps Cicadae*)	*Fungus Sclerotia*	8.33
蝉蜕	*Chántuì* (蟬蛻 *Periostracum Cryptotympanae*)	*Black Cicada Slough*	10.71
蟾酥	*Chánsū* (蟾酥 *Venenum Bufonis*)	*Dried Toads Venom*	10.128

蟾头	*Chántóu* (蟾頭 *Caput Bufinis Sicci*)	*Toad Head*	10.127
辰砂, 朱砂	*Chénshā* (辰砂 *Cinnabaris*)	*Cinnabar*	11.1
沉香	*Chénxiāng* (沉香 *Lignum Aquilariae Resinatum*)	*Chinese eaglewood*	2.46
陈皮	*Chénpí* (陳皮 *Pericarpium Citri Reticulatae*)	*Dried Tangerine Peel*	6.389
赤茯苓	*Chìfúlíng* (赤茯苓 *Poria Rubra*)	*Red Tuckahoe*	8.43
赤芍	*Chìsháo* (赤芍 *Radix Paeoniae Rubra*)	*Red Peony Root*	1.747
赤石脂	*Chìshízhī* (赤石脂 *Halloysitum Rubrum*)	*Red Halloysite*	11.55
赤石脂末	*Chìshízhī* (赤石脂末 *Halloysitum Rubrum*)	*Halloysite*	11.55
川楝子	*Chuānliànzǐ* (川楝子 *Fructus Toosendan*)	*Szechwan Chinaberry Fruit*	6.525
川甜硝, 硝	*Chuāntiánxiāo* (川甜硝 *Natrii Sulfas*)	*Mirabilite*	11.26
川芎	*Chuānxiōng* (川芎 *Rhizoma Chuanxiong*)	*Szechwan Lovage Rhizome*	1.55

(*Continued*)

(Continued)

Simplified Chinese	Pin Yin/Traditional Chinese/Latin Name	Common Name	Zheng Ming Ci Dian Dictionary
大豆黄卷	Dàdòujuǎn (大豆黃卷 Semen Sojae Germinatum)	Germinated Soybean	6.197
大黄	Dàhuáng (大黃 Radix et Rhizoma Rhei Palmati)	Rhubarb Root	1.172
代赭石	Dàizhěshí (代赭石 Haematitum)	Hematite	11.13
胆矾	Dǎnfán (膽礬 Chalcanthitum)	Chalcanthite	11.19
当归	Dāngguī (當歸 Radix Angelicae Sinensis)	Chinese angelica	1.41
灯花	Dēnghuā (燈花 Canglewick)	Wick	
地骨皮	Dìgǔpí (地骨皮 Cortex Lycii Radicis)	Chinese Wolfberry Root-Bark	3.7
地黄	Dìhuáng (地黃 Radix Rehmanniae)	Adhesive Rehmannia Root Tuber	1.763
丁香	Dīngxiāng (丁香 Flos Syzygii Aromatici)	Cloveflower	5.24
定粉，铅粉，宫粉	Dìngfěn (定粉 Lead-Powder)	Lead-Powder	

豆蔻	Dòukòu (豆蔻 *Fructus Amomi Rotundus*)	*Javeamonum Fruit*	6.592
独活	Dúhuó (獨活 *Radix Angelicae Biserratae*)	*Doubleteeth Angelica Root*	1.157
防风	Fángfēng (防風 *Radix Saposhnikoviae*)	*Divaricate Saposhnikovia Root*	1.64
粉霜	Fěnshuāng (粉霜 *Mercury Bichloride*)	*Mercury Bichloride*	
茯苓	Fúlíng (茯苓 *Poria*)	*Indian Buead, Tuckahoe*	8.42
附子	Fùzǐ (附子 *Radix Aconiti Lateralis Preparata*)	*Prepared Common Monkshood Branched Root*	1.639
甘草	Gāncǎo (甘草 *Radix Glycyrrhizae*)	*Liquorice Root*	1.287
甘草炙	Gāncǎo (甘草炙 *Radix Glycyrrhizae Preparata*)	*Liquorice Root*	1.287
甘葛根	Gāngě (甘葛根 *Radix Puerariae Thomsonii*)	*Thomson Kudzuvine Root*	1.314

(Continued)

(Continued)

Simplified Chinese	Pin Yin/Traditional Chinese/Latin Name	Common Name	Zheng Ming Ci Dian Dictionary
甘松	*Gānsōng* (甘松 *Radix et Rhizoma Nardostachyos*)	*Chinese Nardostachys Root and Rhizome*	1.1095
甘遂	*Gānsuì* (甘遂 *Radix Kansui*)	*Gansuiroot, Kansui Root*	1.397
干蟾，蟾	*Gānchán* (幹蟾 *Succy Bufo*)	*Dried Toad*	10.125
干姜	*Gānjiāng* (乾薑 *Rhizoma Zingiberis*)	*Dried Ginger Rhizome*	1.1691
干漆	*Gānqī* (幹漆 *Resina Toxicodendri*)	*Dried Lacquer*	9.39
高良姜	*Gāoliángjiāng* (高良薑 *Rhizoma Alpiniae Officinarum*)	*Lesser Galangal Rhizome*	1.1708
葛根	*Gégēn* (葛根 *Radix Puerariae Lobatae*)	*Lobed Kudzuvine Root*	1.313

钩藤	Gōuténg (钩藤 *Ramulus Uncariae Cum Uncis*)	*Sharpleaf Gambirplant Stem with Hooks*	2.55
瓜蒌	Guālóu (瓜蒌 *Fructus et Semen Trichosanthis*)	*Mongolian Snakegourd Fruit*	6.264
官粉，铅粉	Guānfěn (官粉 *Hydrocerussitum*)	*Lead Carbonate*	11.16
贯众	Guànzhòng (贯众 *Rhizoma Dryopteridis Crassirhizomatis*)	*Male Fern Rhizome*	1.2063
海螵蛸	Hǎipiāoxiāo (海螵蛸 *Endoconcha Sepiellae*)	*Cuttlebone*	10.120
海藻	Hǎizǎo (海藻 *Thallus Sargassi Pallidi*)	*Seaweed*	8.10
寒水石	Hánshuǐshí (寒水石 *Calcitum*)	*Calcite*	11.29
汉防己	Hànfángjǐ (汉防己 *Radix Stephaniae Tetrandrae*)	*Fourstamen Stephania Root*	1.1228
诃子，诃黎勒	Hēzǐ (诃子 *Fructus Chebulae*)	*Medicine Terminalia Fruit*	6.569
鹤虱	Hèshī (鹤虱 *Fructus Carpesii*)	*Common Carpesium Fruit*	6.556

(Continued)

(Continued)

Simplified Chinese	Pin Yin/Traditional Chinese/Latin Name	Common Name	Zheng Ming Ci Dian Dictionary
黑牵牛	Hēiqiānniú (黑牽牛 *Semen Pharbitidis*)	*Lobedleaf Pharbitis Seed*	6.538
黑铅	Hēiqiān (黑鉛)	*Graphite*	
红芽大戟	Hóngyádàjǐ (紅芽大戟 *Knoria valerianoides Thorelet Pitard*)	*Knoxia Corymbosa*	
厚朴	Hòupò (厚樸 *Cortex Magnoliae Officinalis*)	*Officinal Magnolia Bark*	3.84
胡粉, 铅粉, 定粉	Húfěn (胡粉 *Hydrocerussitum*)	*Lead Carbonated*	11.16
胡黄连	Húhuánglián (胡黃連 *Rhizoma Picrorhizae*)	*Figwort flower Picrorhiza Rhizome*	1.783
胡椒	Hújiāo (胡椒 *Fructus Piperis Nigri*)	*Black Pepper Fruit*	6.364
虎杖	Hǔzhàng (虎杖 *Rhizoma Polygoni Cuspidati*)	*Giant Knotweed Rhizome*	1.208
琥珀	Hǔpò (琥珀 *Succinum*)	*Amber*	11.70

滑石	Huáshí (滑石 Talcum)	Talc	11.63
怀山药, 山药	Huáishānyào (懷山藥 Rhizoma Dioscoreae Oppositae)	Common Yam Rhizome	1.1909
黄柏	Huángbǎi (黃柏 Cortex Phellodendri Amurensis)	Amur Corktree Bark	3.208
黄蝉壳	Huángchánké (黃蟬殼 Periostracum Cicadae)	Cicada Slough	10.71
黄丹,铅丹	Huángdān (黃丹 Minium)	Lead Oxide	11.15
黄瓜	Huángguā (黃瓜 Fructus Cucumis Sativi)	Cucumber	6.313
黄连	Huánglián (黃連 Rhizoma Coptidis)	Chinese Goldthread	1.593
黄明胶	Huángmíngjiāo (黃明膠 Collacorii Bovis)	Oxhide Gelatin	10.227
黄芩	Huángqín (黃芩 Radix Scutellariae Baicalensis)	Baikal Skullcap Root	1.1320
藿香	Huòxiāng (藿香 Herba Agastaches Rugosae)	Wrinkled Gianthyssop Herb	7.724

(Continued)

(Continued)

Simplified Chinese	Pin Yin/Traditional Chinese/Latin Name	Common Name	Zheng Ming Ci Dian Dictionary
鸡舌香，母丁香	Jīshéxiāng (雞舌香 Fructus Syzygii Aromatici)	Clove Fruit	6.3
浆水	Jiāngshuǐ (漿水)	Malting Liquid	
金箔	Jīnbó (金箔)	Native Gold	
金星石，金精石	Jīnxīngshí (金星石 Vermiculitum)	Vermiculite	11.67
金银花	Jīnyínhuā (金銀花 Flos Lonicerae)	Japanese Honeysuckle Flower Bud	5.83
荆芥	Jīngjiè (荊芥 Herba Schizonepetae Tenuifoliae)	Fineleaf Schizonepeta Herb	7.823
粳米	Jīngmǐ (粳米 Semen Oryzae Sativae)	Rice	6.629
桔梗	Jiégěng (桔梗 Radix Platycodi)	Balloonflower Root	1.469

橘皮, 陈皮	Júpí (橘皮 *Pericarpium Citri Reticulatae*)	*Tangerine Peel*	6.389
苦楝皮, 苦楝根皮	Kǔliàngēnpí (苦楝皮 *Cortex Meliae Azedarach*)	*Chinaberry-Tree Bark*	3.128
苦杏仁	Kǔxìngrén (苦杏仁 *Semen Armeniacae Amarum*)	*Ansu Apricot Seed*	6.40
栝蒌根	Guālóugēn (栝蒌根 *Fructus*)	*Snakegourd Fruit*	6.264
腊茶	Làchá (臘茶)	*Winter Tea*	
兰香叶, 兰香	Lánxiāng (蘭香葉 *Herba seu Radix Caryopteridis Incanae*)	*Common Bluebeard Herb*	7.943
雷丸	Léiwán (雷丸 *Omphalia*)	*Stone-Like Omphalia*	8.40
羚羊角	Língyángjiǎo (羚羊角 *Cornu Saigae Tataricae*)	*Antelope Horn*	10.186
硫黄	Liúhuáng (硫黄 *Sulfur*)	*Sulphur*	11.50
龙齿	Lóngchǐ (龍齒 *Dens Draconis*)	*Dragon's Teeth*	11.74
龙骨	Lónggǔ (龍骨 *Os Draconis*)	*Dragon's Bones*	11.73

(*Continued*)

(Continued)

Simplified Chinese	Pin Yin/Traditional Chinese/Latin Name	Common Name	Zheng Ming Ci Dian Dictionary
龙脑, 冰片	Lóngnǎo (龍腦 *Borneolum Syntheticum*)	*Borneol*	9.27
芦荟	Lúhuì (蘆薈 *Aloe*)	*Aloe*	9.5
萝卜根	Luóbogēn (蘿蔔根 *Radux Raphani Sativi*)	*Garden Radish*	6.341
萝卜子, 莱服子	Luóbozǐ (蘿蔔子 *Semen Raphani Sativi*)	*Gardon Raddish Seed*	6.341
绿豆	Lǜdòu (綠豆 *Semen Vignae Radiatae*)	*Mung Bean*	6.206
绿矾	Lǜfán (綠礬 *Melanteritum*)	*Green Vitriol*	11.11
麻黄	Máhuáng (麻黃 *Herba Ephedrae Sinicae*)	*Chinese Ephedra Herb*	7.1565
马兜铃	Mǎdōulíng (馬兜鈴 *Fructus Aristolochiae Debilis*)	*Slender Dutchmanspipe Fruit*	6.11
马牙硝, 芒硝	Mǎyáxiāo (馬牙硝 *Natrii Sulfas*)	*Mirabilite*	11.26

麦门冬, 麦冬	*Màidōng* (麥門冬 *Radix Ophiopogonis Japonici*)	*Dwarf Lilyturf Root Tuber*	1.1778
没石子, 没食子	*Mòishízi* (沒石子 *Galla Turcica*)	*Gallnut*	9.43
米泔	*Mǐgān* (米泔 *Rice-Washed Water*)	*Rice-Washed Water*	
墨, 好墨	*Mò* (好墨 *Inkstick*)	*Inkstick*	
牡丹皮	*Mǔdānpí* (牡丹皮 *Cortex Moutan Radicis*)	*Tree Peony Root-Bark*	3.1
牡蛎	*Mǔlì* (牡蠣 *Concha Ostreae*)	*Common Oyster Shell*	10.28
木瓜	*Mùguā* (木瓜 *Fructus Chaenomelis Sprciosae*)	*Common Floweringquince Fruit*	6.24
木通	*Mùtōng* (木通 *Caulis Akebiae*)	*Akabia Stem*	2.110
木香	*Mùxiāng* (木香 *Radix Aucklandiae*)	*Costusroot, Common Aucklandia Root*	1.875

(*Continued*)

(Continued)

Simplified Chinese	Pin Yin/Traditional Chinese/Latin Name	Common Name	Zheng Ming Ci Dian Dictionary
木香, 南木香	*Mùxiāng* (木香 *Radix Aristolochiae*)	*Costustroot, Common Aucklandia Root*	1.875
硇砂	*Náoshā* (硇砂 *Sal Ammoniac*)	*Ammonium Chloride*	11.38
脑子, 樟脑	*Nǎozi* (腦子 *Camphora*)	*Camphor*	9.12
腻粉, 轻粉	*Nìfěn* (腻粉 *Calomelas*) *Qīngfěn* (輕粉 *Calomelas*)	*Calomel*	11.5
牛胆	*Niúdǎn* (牛膽 *Fel Bovis*)	*Ox Galbladderl*	10.220
牛黄	*Niúhuáng* (牛黄 *Calculus Bovis*)	*Cow Bezoar*	10.223
牛李子	*Niúlǐzǐ* (牛李子 *Fructus Rhamnni Davuricae*)	*Davurian Buckthorn Fruit*	6.355
糯稻根须	*Nuòdàogēnxū* (糯稻根須 *Radix Oryzae Glutinosae*)	*Stichy Rice Root*	1.2026

糯米	Nuòmǐ (糯米 Oryzae Glutinosae)	Glutinous Rice	1.2026
硼砂	Péngshā (硼砂 Borax)	Borax	11.49
坏子胭脂，干胭脂	Pīzǐyānzhī (坏子胭脂 Dactylopius Coccus Costa)	Dried Carmine	
砒霜	Pīshuāng (砒霜 Arsenicum Sublimatum)	Arsenic	11.47
蒲扇灰	Púshànhuī (蒲扇灰)	Ash of Cattail Leaf Fan	
牵牛子，黑白牵牛	Qiānniúzǐ (牵牛 Semen Pharbitidis)	Lobedleaf Pharbitis Seed	6.538
铅丹	Qiāndān (铅丹 Plumbum Rubrum)	Lead Oxside	11.15
前胡	Qiánhú (前胡 Radix Peucedani)	Whiteflower Hogfennel Root	1.82
芡实 (鸡头)	Qiànshí (芡實 Semen Euryales)	Gordon Euryale Seed	6.499
羌活	Qiānghuó (羌活 Rhizoma et Radix Notopterygii)	Incised Notopterygium Rhizome	1.151

(*Continued*)

(Continued)

Simplified Chinese	Pin Yin/Traditional Chinese/Latin Name	Common Name	Zheng Ming Ci Dian Dictionary
秦艽	*Qínjiāo* (秦艽 *Radix Gentianae Macrophyllae*)	*Largeleaf Gentian Root*	1.437
秦皮	*Qínpí* (秦皮 *Cortex Fraxini*)	*Ash Bark*	3.113
青黛	*Qīngdài* (青黛 *Indigo Naturalis*)	*Natural Indigo*	9.28
青蛤粉, 青黛	*Qīnggéfěn* (青蛤粉 *Indigo Naturalis*)	*Natural Indigo*	9.28
青橘皮, 青皮	*Qīngpí* (青橘皮 *Fructus Citri Reticulatae Immaturus*)	*Green Tangerine Peel*	6.391
青礞石	*Qīngméngshí* (青礞石 *Lapis Chloriti*)	*Biotite Schist*	11.65
轻粉, 腻粉	*Qīngfěn* (輕粉 *Calomelas*)	*Calomel*	11.5
全蝎	*Quánxiē* (全蠍 *Scorpio*)	*Scorpion*	10.94
人参	*Rénshēn* (人参 *Radix Ginseng*)	*Ginseng*	1.1

肉豆蔻	Ròudòukòu (肉豆蔻 *Semen Myristicae*)	*Nutmeg*	6.320
肉桂	Ròuguì (肉桂 *Cortex Cinnamomi/Cassiae*)	*Cassia Bark*	3.185
桑白皮	Sāngbáipí (桑白皮 *Cortex Mori Albae Radicis*)	*White Mulberry Root-Bark*	3.145
砂仁	Shārén (砂仁 *Fructus Amomi*)	*Villous Amomum Fruit*	6.578
山栀	Shānzhī (山栀 *Fructus Gardeniae*)	*Cape Jasmine Fruit*	6.173
山茱萸	Shānzhūyú (山茱萸 *Fructus Corni*)	*Asiatic Cornelian Cherry Fruit*	6.1
芍药	Sháoyào (芍药 *Radix Paeoniae Alba*)	*White Peony Root*	1.746
蛇黄, 蛇含石	Shéhuáng (蛇黄 *Pyritum Globuloforme*)	*Globular Pyrite*	11.9
麝香	Shèxiāng (麝香 *Moschus*)	*Forest Musk*	10.241
升麻	Shēngmá (升麻 *Rhizoma Cimicifugae Foetidae*)	*Skunk Bugbane Rhizome*	1.735
升药	Shēngyào (升药 *Hydrargyri Oxydatum Rubrum*)	*Red Oxide of Mexcury*	11.6

(Continued)

(Continued)

Simplified Chinese	Pin Yin/Traditional Chinese/Latin Name	Common Name	Zheng Ming Ci Dian Dictionary
生地	Shēngdì (生地 Radix Rehmanniae)	Adhesive Rehmannia Root Tuber	1.763
生姜	Shēngjiāng (生薑 Rhizoma Zingiberis Recens)	Fresh Ginger	1.1690
生犀	Shēngxī (生犀 Cornu Rhinoceri Asiatici)	Rhinoceros Horn	
石膏	Shígāo (石膏 Gypsum Fibrosum)	Gypsum	11.21
石斛	Shíhú (石斛 Herba Dendrobii Nobilis)	Noble Dendrobium Stem Herb	7.1374
石榴根皮	Shíliúgēnpí (石榴根皮 Cortex Granati Radicis)	Granati Root Bark	
石榴皮	Shíliúpí (石榴皮 Pericarpium Punicae Granati)	Pome Granate Rind	6.8

石脑油	Shínǎoyóu (石腦油 Petroleum Naphtha Ligroin)	Naphtha	
使君子	Shǐjūnzǐ (使君子 Fructus Quisqualis)	Rangooncreeper Fruit	6.567
黍粘子	Shǔzhānzǐ (黍粘子 Semen Panici Miliacei)	Broomcorn Millet	
水牛角	Shuǐniújiǎo (水牛角 CornuBubali)	Buffalo Horn	10.218
水银	Shuǐyín (水銀 Hydrargyrum)	Mercury	11.2
松子仁肉	Sōngzǐrén (松子仁肉 Pinus Pinea)	Pine Nut	6.643
桃枝	Táozhī (桃枝 Ramulus Persicae)	Peach Twig	2.156
天麻	Tiānmá (天麻 Rhizoma Gastrodiae)	Tall Gastrodis Rhizome	1.1950
天门冬	Tiānméndōng (天門冬 Radix Asparagi Cochinchinensis)	Cochinchinese Asparagus Root	1.1795
天南星, 炙天南星	Tiānnánxīng (炙天南星 Rhizoma Arisaematis)	Jack-In-The-Pulpit Tuber	1.1621

(Continued)

(Continued)

Simplified Chinese	Pin Yin/Traditional Chinese/Latin Name	Common Name	Zheng Ming Ci Dian Dictionary
天台乌药	*Tiāntái Wūyào* (天臺烏藥 *Radix Linderae Aggregatae*)	*Combined Spicebush Root*	1.1251
天竹黄	*Tiānzhúhuáng* (天竹黃 *Concretio Silicea Bambusae*)	*Tabasheer*	9.14
天竺黄	*Tiānzhúhuáng* (天竺黃 *Concretio Silicea Bambusae*)	*Tabasheer*	9.14
甜瓜蒂, 瓜蒂	*Tiánguādì* (甜瓜蒂 *Pedicellus Melo*)	*Muskmelon Base*	6.312
甜硝, 川甜硝	*Tiánxiāo* (甜硝 *Sweet Mirabilite*)	*Sweet Mirabilite*	
甜杏仁	*Tiánxìngrén* (甜杏仁 *Semen Armeniacae Dulce*)	*Common Apricot Seed*	6.39
铁粉	*Tiěfěn* (鐵粉 *Ferrous Pulveres*)	*Iron Powder*	
葶苈, 甜葶苈, 葶苈子	*Tínglì* (葶藶 *Semen LepidiiApetali*)	*Pepperweed Seed*	6.331

铜青，铜绿	*Tóngqīng* (銅青 *Mineralium Viridianum*)	*Verdigris*	11.68
乌梅	*Wūméi* (烏梅 *Fructus Mume*)	*Smoked Plum*	6.38
乌梢蛇，乌蛇肉	*Wūshāoshé* (烏梢蛇 *Zaocys*)	*Black Snake*	10.146
乌药	*Wūyào* (烏藥 *Radix Linderae Aggregatae*)	*Combined Spicebush Root*	1.1251
蜈蚣	*Wúgōng* (蜈蚣 *Scolopendra*)	*Centipede*	10.95
芜荑，白芜荑	*Wúyí* (蕪荑 *Pasta Ulmi*)	*Bigfruit Elm Pasdt*	9.33
五灵脂	*Wǔlíngzhī* (五靈脂 *Faeces Trogopterori*)	*Trogopterus Dung*	10.170
虾蟆，虾蟆灰，干虾蟆	*Xiāmá* (蝦蟆 *Rana Siccus*)	*Dried Chinese Woodfrog*	10.131
香附	*Xiāngfù* (香附 *Rhizoma Cyperi*)	*Nutgrass Galingale Rhizome*	1.2030

(Continued)

(Continued)

Simplified Chinese	Pin Yin/Traditional Chinese/Latin Name	Common Name	Zheng Ming Ci Dian Dictionary
硝，芒硝	*Xiāo* (芒硝 *Natrii Sulfas*)	*Mirabilite*	11.26
蝎尾，全蝎	*Xiēwěi* (蠍尾 *Cauda Scorpionis*)	*Scorpion*	10.94
杏仁	*Xìngrén* (杏仁 *Semen Armeniacae Amarum*)	*Bitter Apricot Seed*	6.60
熊胆	*Xióngdǎn* (熊膽 *Fel Selenarcti*)	*Bear Gall Bladder*	10.215
雄黄	*Xiónghuáng* (雄黃 *Realgar*)	*Redopiment*	11.52
续随子	*Xùsuízi* (續隨子 *Semen Euphorbia lathyris*)	*Moleweed*	6.183
玄参	*Xuánshēn* (玄參 *Radix Scrophulariae*)	*Figwort Root*	1.759
玄精石	*Xuánjīngshí* (玄精石 *Selenitum*)	*Selenite*	11.23
胭脂花	*Yānzhīhuā* (胭脂花 *Primula Maximowiczii*)	*Carmine Flowers*	
延胡索	*Yánhúsuǒ* (延胡索 *Rhizoma Corydalis*)	*Yanghusuo Tuber*	1.798
羊子肝	*Yángzǐgān* (羊子肝 *Jecur Caprae*)	*Goat Liver*	10.198
夜明砂	*Yèmíngshā* (夜明砂 *Faeces Vespertilionis*)	*Bat Feces*	10.172
银星石	*Yínxīngshí* (銀星石 *Wavellite*)	*Wavellite*	

榆仁	*Yúrén (榆仁 Semen Ulmi Pumilae)*	*Dwarf Elm Seed*	
禹余粮	*Yǔyúliáng (禹餘糧 Limonitum)*	*Limonite*	11.8
郁金	*Yùjīn (郁金 Radix Curcumae Wenyujin)*	*Wenchow Turmeric Root Tuber*	1.1697
郁李仁	*Yùlǐrén (郁李仁 Semen Pruni Japonicae)*	*Chinese Bushcherry Seed*	6.51
枣	*Zǎo (棗 Fructus Jujubae)*	*Common Jujube*	6.351
皂荚子	*Zàojiázǐ (皂莢子 Semen Gleditsiae Sinensis)*	*Chinese Honeylocust Seed*	6.251
泽泻	*Zéxiè (澤瀉 Rhizoma Alismatis)*	*Oriental Waterplantain Rhizome Tuber*	1.1604
珍珠	*Zhēnzhū (珍珠 Margarita)*	*Pearl*	10.36
知母	*Zhīmǔ (知母 Rhizoma Anemarrhenae)*	*Common Anemarrhena*	1.1776
枳壳	*Zhǐqiào (枳殼 Fructus Aurantii Submatures)*	*Submature Bitter Orange*	6.371

(Continued)

(Continued)

Simplified Chinese	Pin Yin/Traditional Chinese/Latin Name	Common Name	Zheng Ming Ci Dian Dictionary
积实	*Zhǐshí* (积實 *Fructus Aurantii Immaturus*)	*Immature Bitter Orange*	6.370
猪胆粉, 猪胆	*Zhūdǎnfěn* (豬膽粉 *Pulvis Fellis Suis*)	*Pig Gall Powder*	
猪胆汁	*Zhūdǎnzhī* (豬膽汁 *Fel Suillus*)	*Pig Bile*	10.207
猪粪	*Zhūfèn* (豬糞 *Pig Manure*)	*Pig Manure*	
猪悬蹄甲	*Zhūtíjiǎ* (豬懸蹄甲)	*Pig Hoof Nail*	
竹叶	*Zhúyè* (竹葉 *Olium Phyllostachytis Henonis*)	*Henon Bamboo Leaf*	4.203
紫草	*Zǐcǎo* (紫草 *Radix Lithospermi*)	*Redroot Gromwell Root*	1.242
紫草茸	*Zǐcǎoróng* (紫草茸 *Lacca*)	*Shellac*	10.96
紫苏	*Zǐsū* (紫蘇 *Folium Perillae Zugutae*)	*Perilla Leaf*	

Printed in the United States
By Bookmasters